Supporting Positive Behaviour

Knowledge and Skills for Social Care Workers series

The *Knowledge and Skills for Social Care Workers* series features accessible and interactive open learning workbooks which tackle a range of key subjects relevant to people working with adults in residential or domiciliary settings. Topics covered in this series include how social care workers can communicate effectively, health and safety, safeguarding adults from harm and abuse and supporting relationships and friendships.

other books in the series

Supporting Relationships and Friendships
A Workbook for Social Care Workers
Suzan Collins
ISBN 978 1 84905 072 2

Effective Communication
A Workbook for Social Care Workers
Suzan Collins
ISBN 978 1 84310 027 3

Safeguarding Adults
A Workbook for Social Care Workers
Suzan Collins
ISBN 978 1 84310 928 0

Health and Safety
A Workbook for Social Care Workers
Suzan Collins
ISBN 978 1 84310 929 7

Reflecting On and Developing Your Practice
A Workbook for Social Care Workers
Suzan Collins
ISBN 978 1 84310 930 3

Supporting Positive Behaviour

A Workbook for Social Care Workers

Suzan Collins

Jessica Kingsley Publishers
London and Philadelphia

First published in 2010
by Jessica Kingsley Publishers
116 Pentonville Road
London N1 9JB, UK
and
400 Market Street, Suite 400
Philadelphia, PA 19106, USA

www.jkp.com

Copyright © Suzan Collins 2010

All rights reserved. No part of this publication may be reproduced in any material form (including photocopying or storing it in any medium by electronic means and whether or not transiently or incidentally to some other use of this publication) without the written permission of the copyright owner except in accordance with the provisions of the Copyright, Designs and Patents Act 1988 or under the terms of a licence issued by the Copyright Licensing Agency Ltd, Saffron House, 6–10 Kirby Street, London EC1N 8TS. Applications for the copyright owner's written permission to reproduce any part of this publication should be addressed to the publisher.

Warning: The doing of an unauthorised act in relation to a copyright work may result in both a civil claim for damages and criminal prosecution.

All pages marked ✓ may be photocopied for personal use with this programme, but may not be reproduced for any other purposes without the permission of the publisher

Library of Congress Cataloging in Publication Data
A CIP catalog record for this book is available from the Library of Congress

British Library Cataloguing in Publication Data
A CIP catalogue record for this book is available from the British Library

ISBN 978 1 84905 073 9

Printed and bound by
MPG Books Limited

Acknowledgements

I would like to thank the following people for their advice and support:

Alison Mallett, Assistant Practitioner Social Service

Janet Elliott, Safeguarding Adults Lead, Suffolk, Primary Care Trust

Karen Patterson, KP Social Training Ltd

Robert Baines (Home Farm Trust) for providing a copy of a risk assessment form and information on risk assessment, risk management and risk communication

Samantha Cable and Lauren Dowsing, for letting me photograph them and using the photographs for this workbook

Thank you to Ian Julian for his support

Maslow's Hierarchy of Needs, p.64: all reasonable efforts to trace the copyright holder have been made, and any queries should be addressed to the publishers.

This workbook meets the requirements of the following standards, guidance and qualifications:

Care Quality Commission (CQC)
Care Home for Adults Standards 6, 7 and 23
Care Home for Older People Standard 18
Domiciliary Standards 7 and 12

General Social Care Council (GSCC)
Code of Practice Standard 4

Skills for Care (SfC)
Common Induction Standard (CIS) 1

Contents

Introduction	9
Responsibilities	12
What is Behaviour?	15
Causes of Challenging Behaviour	17
Reacting and Responding to Challenging Behaviour	34
Self-Harm	42
How to Minimize and/or Prevent Challenging Behaviour	45
The Principles of Care: Respecting Service Users with Challenging Behaviour	71
Health, Safety and Risk	78
Reporting and Recording	86
Taking Care of Yourself and Being Supported	98
Self-Assessment Tool	106
Certificate	107
Legislation and Useful Websites	109
References and Further Reading	111

Introduction

SUPPORTING PEOPLE WITH THEIR BEHAVIOUR

This workbook will help you to understand some of the causes and reasons why people might show what appears to be challenging behaviour and how you might reduce its incidence. You must respect each service user and provide the same level of care and support to each individual, regardless of whether or not they are presenting challenging behaviour.

The General Social Care Council (GSCC) has devised a set of standards that your employer and you as a social care worker should work within. Respecting service users and providing each individual with the same care are both required by the standards. The standards contain good practice and professional conduct requirements. There are six standards and you can find out the contents of each standard by obtaining a copy of the Codes of Practice from your manager or, if you are recently in post, then you should have received a copy of the booklet in your induction pack. Alternatively, you can access a copy on the GSCC website (www.gscc.org.uk). You will learn about the contents of Standard 4, entitled 'Respect the rights of service users while seeking to ensure that their behaviour does not harm themselves or other people', later in the book (p.79).

This respect should be for everyone regardless of their age, abilities or needs, for example people with a learning and/or physical disability, or people with dementia, older people and people with mental health needs, whether or not they have challenging behaviour.

During my career I have often been asked about working with people who show challenging behaviour: how I could work with 'those people' and told 'it should be strong and muscular men who should work with them'. I would reply that it is not about strength, it is about communicating and using tested techniques to enrich the lives of the people with whom you work.

Who are the right people to support those with challenging behaviour? I would say people with a caring and supportive nature who are willing to undergo training and see the service user as a person with needs, rights and wishes.

ABOUT THIS BOOK

It is not always possible for staff to be taken off the rota to attend a training course and so this workbook has been devised. It uses a variety of training methods:

- reading passages where you will expand your knowledge
- completing exercises
- completing a self-assessment tool which shows you the knowledge you have acquired.

As a social care worker, you have to work to certain standards, which are set out by various professional bodies. This workbook links to several standards and in case you are not familiar with them, here is a brief explanation of each one.

Skills for Care (SfC) has a set of standards called Common Induction Standards which apply to all new staff in the care sector (except those who are supporting people with learning disabilities, who will need to complete the Learning Disability Qualification Induction Award). The Common Induction Standards and the Learning Disability Qualification Induction Award should be completed within three months of being in post. This workbook meets the requirements of the Common Induction Standard 1.

Care Quality Commission (CQC) took over the work of the Commission for Social Care Inspection (CSCI) on 1 April 2009 (it also took over the work of the Healthcare Commission and the Mental Health Act Commission). The CQC has sets of standards for you and your workplace to meet. There are different sets of standards and it will depend on where you work as to which standards you need to work to. If you are unsure, please ask your manager. This workbook meets the requirements of Care Home for Adults Standards 6, 7 and 23, Care Home for Older People Standard 18 and the Domiciliary Care Standards 7 and 12; references to these standards are made in this workbook.

General Social Care Council (GSCC) has a Code of Practice with six standards that reflect good practice. This workbook meets the requirements of Standard 4 and reference to this standard is made in this workbook.

Towards the end of the workbook you will be asked to complete a self-assessment questionnaire on what you have learnt from completing this workbook. Once you have completed this, your manager or trainer will complete the certificate on pp. 104–105 and give it to you. You will then have completed training on managing challenging behaviour.

I hope that you find this a useful workbook and wish you well in your career.

This workbook can be:

- read straight through from front to back
- used as a reference book.

In this workbook, I have referred to the people you support as 'service users' and 'he/him' rather than continually writing he/she or him/her.

Name of Learner: ....

Signature of Learner: .... Date:. ....

Name of Manager or Trainer: ....

Signature of Manager or Trainer: .... Date:. ....

Workplace address or name of organization:

....

....

....

....

Responsibilities

Everyone who is supporting a person with challenging behaviour in the care setting has responsibilities, and it will depend on the position the person holds as to what their responsibilities are.

MANAGERS' RESPONSIBILITIES

Social care employers must:

- Make sure people are suitable to enter the workforce and understand their roles and responsibilities;
- Have written policies and procedures in place to enable social care workers to meet the General Social Care Council (GSCC) Code of Practice for Social Care Workers;
- Provide training and development opportunities to enable social care workers to strengthen and develop their skills and knowledge;
- Put in place and implement written policies and procedures to deal with dangerous, discriminatory or exploitative behaviour and practice; and
- Promote the GSCC's code of practice to social care workers, service users and carers and co-operate with the GSCC's proceedings. (GSCC 2002)

Social care employers must provide written guidance and this will be in the form of:

- care plans or support plans
- risk assessments
- guidance on what to do if a service user is challenging.

You will read more about these as you progress through this workbook.

Social care managers are responsible for liaising with other professionals, including general practitioners (GPs), Social Services, Drugs and Alcohol team, police and Probation. There are different processes in place in each of these areas.

SOCIAL CARE WORKERS' RESPONSIBILITIES

General Social Care Council Standard 4:
Social care workers must:

- As a social care worker, you must respect the rights of service users while seeking to ensure that their behaviour does not harm themselves or other people.
- Recognizing that service users have the right to take risks and helping them to identify and manage potential and actual risks to themselves and others;
- Following risk assessment polices and procedures to assess whether the behaviour of service users presents a risk of harm to themselves or others;
- Taking necessary steps to minimize the risks of service users from doing actual or potential harm to themselves or other people; and
- Ensuring that relevant colleagues and agencies are informed about the outcomes and implications of risk assessments. (GSCC 2002)

As a social care worker, you should:

- follow your job description
- read, understand and follow policies, procedures and risk assessments (you will read more about risk assessments on pp.78–83)
- promote the rights of the people you support
- understand positive risk taking
- implement the principles of care
- be open and friendly and do not prejudge as it is not the service user's fault that he is using behaviour to tell you something.

✎ How do your organization's policies and procedures on managing behaviour affect what you do?

....
....
....
....

SERVICE USERS' RESPONSIBILITIES

Service users should:

- avoid knowingly putting themselves and/or others at risk
- contribute wherever possible to their risk assessment and work with services to reduce and minimize risks.

What is Behaviour?

An example of an action that can be classed as behaviour is walking along the street.

> Behaviour has to be:
> - observable
> - measurable
> - describable.
>
> It is what we can see others (and ourselves) doing.

An example of an action that cannot be classed as behaviour is feeling lonely.

WHAT IS CHALLENGING BEHAVIOUR?

Challenging behaviour is 'culturally abnormal behaviour of such intensity, frequency or duration that the person or others are likely to be placed in serious jeopardy or behaviour which is likely to seriously limit or delay access to and use of ordinary community facilities' (Emerson 1995, p.3).

Some examples of behaviour that you may find challenging:

- physical aggression
- self-stimulation
- damage to property
- reckless disregard for the safety of yourself or another.

✍ Please tick [✓] the types of behaviour that you have seen happen in your workplace:

Behaviour	✓
Hitting	
Punching	
Biting	
Slapping	
Throwing furniture	
Shouting	
Swearing	
Hair-pulling	
Sitting still, being withdrawn and not interacting	
Self-harm: this might be a person cutting, burning, scalding, banging or scratching their own body, pulling their hair, breaking their bones, or ingesting toxic substances or objects (more information on self-harm can be found on p.42–44)	
Other:	

> When you see challenging behaviour, you must not punish the service user for the behaviour being shown.

Causes of Challenging Behaviour

Service users present many different kinds of challenging behaviour, for a variety of reasons. Here are some examples:

- difficulties in communicating
- stress
- environmental causes
- reacting to staff
- reacting to parents or relatives
- feeling physically unwell
- feeling sad or angry
- experiences of loss and change
- feelings of low self-esteem
- nature (individuals' innate qualities) or nurture (personal experiences) problems.

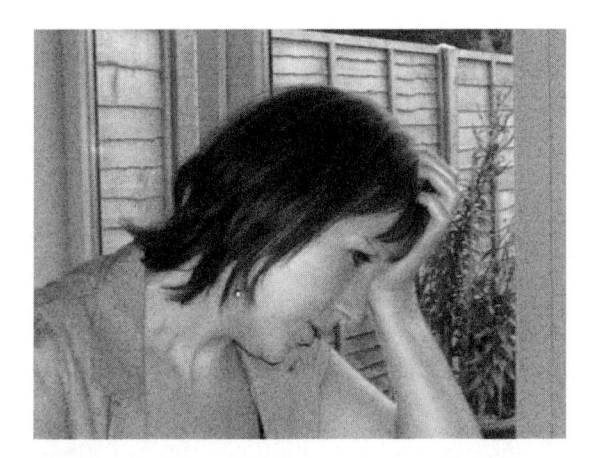

Feeling stressed

DIFFICULTIES IN COMMUNICATING

Communication is important for all of us as it helps us to be in control of our own lives. If we cannot communicate, we will end up in a position where someone else controls our life for us, because we cannot say what we want and need.

> Staff provide service users with the information, assistance and communication support they need to make decisions about their own lives. (CQC Care Home for Adults Standard 7.2)

When people show challenging behaviour, they are trying to communicate with you in their unique way. For example, John might bang his cup on the table to indicate he has finished the drink or would like a drink, while Jane might tap her forehead twice to indicate that she would like a drink. You will need to get to know each service user to find out each person's unique way of communicating: some can be straightforward, some are not.

It is important that you learn how to communicate with the service user and in a way that is appropriate to him, so that person can comment and express his views, needs and wishes. It may be necessary for you to teach the service user skills to enable him to communicate with others. There is more guidance on how to do this in the workbook *Effective Communication* which is also published in this series.

Why we communicate

We communicate for a variety of reasons. It might be:

- to get a message across
- to express thoughts and feelings
- to feel and be included
- to get to know people
- to be in control.

How we communicate

Communication can be observed in many ways. Perhaps the most obvious form that people think about is verbally, but other important forms of communication include *body language*, such as smiling to show you are happy, or dropping your head and frowning to show you are unhappy. It can also be observed in your *actions*: for example, clapping your hands to show you are happy, or slamming a door or throwing a cup to show that you are unhappy.

> If you smile, the other person will smile back.
> If you look grumpy, the other person will more than likely ignore you.

Here is an exercise you may like to try. It will enable you to experience what it is like to be unable to express yourself verbally.

✍ You want a cup of tea but you cannot talk as you have lost your voice, and your leg is in plaster so you cannot walk to the kitchen and make it yourself. Because you have no voice, you cannot let others know what you want.

How do you feel?

....
....
....
....

I guess some of your answers may include: thirsty, angry and frustrated.

> Remember: if you cannot communicate with the service user and he cannot communicate with you, it will be very difficult for him to make choices and become or remain independent, and it is more likely that he will present challenging behaviour. More information can be found in the workbook on *Effective Communication*.

Communicating and being assertive

We are not born assertive, we have to learn it, which usually means training. Another way is to watch others who are assertive and then practise it ourselves. The people you support will see you as role models and may copy what you do.

If you are an assertive person you can be described as self-assured and confident, and this will reflect in how you put your message across with confidence. You can say 'No' to a request without becoming controlling. However, there is a difference between being assertive and being aggressive. If you are an aggressive person, you may find yourself described by others as forceful, hostile, sulky, sarcastic, getting your own way by upsetting others in whichever way works for you.

If a service user cannot put his message across in an assertive manner it can be interpreted as aggressive and this can result in others ignoring him, arguing, shouting, being abrupt, people not listening to him or walking away when he is trying to communicate.

✎ There are classes available to learn to be assertive.

Would any of the people you support benefit from learning this? Yes/No
If you have answered 'Yes', what are you going to do about it?

....
....
....
....

> **Being careful how you communicate: the power of words**
>
> The words you use can affect how people are respected, and are powerful things. For example, if you were to say 'I will allow the service user to…', you are asserting your control over the people you support. Instead, staff should *enable* the service user to do things. Staff should not 'allow', as it is the service user who should be in control.

✎ Think of an occasion when a service user had challenging behaviour. What was the reason for this and what did you do?

....
....
....
....

Communicating through behaviour

Here are some examples of how behaviour can be used to try to tell you something.

Actions	Possible reason
Smiling when a particular member of staff walks through the front door	The service user likes that member of staff.
Clapping hands and laughing	The service user is happy.
Standing too close to someone, and so appearing aggressive and intimidating	Different cultures have different norms on what is acceptable for personal space: the service user may simply be behaving normally.
Throwing a cup	Thirst: would the service user like a drink?
Repeating the word 'sausage' over and over again	The service user may want sausages for tea, hate sausages, or perhaps they have just learnt to say this word.
Screaming when a particular person is near by	They may not like this person.
Taking off clothes in an inappropriate place, such as the middle of the lounge	This could be telling you that the clothes are too tight, that he wants to wear different clothes, or that he would like a bath.
Hitting other people	Is the service user in pain, upset or angry? Think about what might have made him so.
Getting up and wandering around in the night	Perhaps the service user used to live at home and shared a double bed with a partner, and now finds it difficult sleeping alone in a small single bed.

✎ Imagine that you have just won the lottery. What is your behaviour like?

....
....
....
....

I guess you may have been: smiling, laughing, jumping up and down with excitement, and rushing to the telephone to tell others of your good news.

SUPPORTING POSITIVE BEHAVIOUR

✎ Imagine now that you have a headache. You have no speech and no other means to let the staff know that you have a headache e.g. no writing paper and pen and they are not looking in your direction anyway. How does this make you feel?

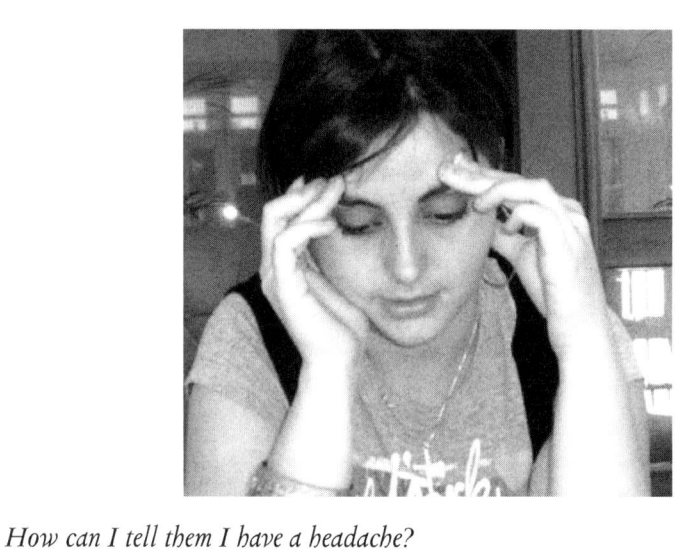

How can I tell them I have a headache?

....
....
....
....

How will you tell others that you have a headache?

....
....
....
....

Was challenging behaviour involved?   Yes/No

Was your behaviour out of character for you?   Yes/No

CAUSES OF CHALLENGING BEHAVIOUR

What would other people say if they saw you doing what you did?

....
....
....
....

LABELLING BEHAVIOUR

In the future, people may remember the day you had a headache as the day you got upset or angry, but they may never know why.

This can happen with some people you support, and if it does, it can lead to people thinking of them as having a tendency to present challenging behaviour. When this happens, people can focus on the challenging behaviour rather than a person who is good at most things but can become distressed or frustrated when he cannot communicate how he feels. It is important that people who express themselves through challenging behaviour are not discriminated against because of the behaviour they are showing while communicating.

LABELS

People who express themselves through behaviour can be labelled as 'difficult' or 'having challenging behaviour'.

✎ Is it fair to give someone a label because he cannot communicate verbally or he has not been given the tools (e.g. pictures or photographs) to communicate and express his needs? Yes/No

Please explain your answer:

....
....
....
....

If someone is given a label, carers may see the label before seeing the person as a human being with needs, rights and wishes. They may tend to want to stop the behaviour before getting to know the person and understand why the behaviour is there, or avoid the service user altogether.

✍ Think of one of the people you support. Without revealing the person's name, write down four things about them:

1. ....

2. ....

3. ....

4. ....

Now look back at your answers. Did you write down mostly positive or negative things about the service user?   Positive/Negative

✍ If you wrote down negative things, what can you do to change them to positive?

....

....

....

....

The effects of giving service users a negative label can include the following:

- giving carers low expectations of them and the service user feeling no need to rise to challenges
- giving the service user a low sense of self-esteem
- providing the service user with fewer chances in life, which can lead to missed opportunities in developing.

The effects of giving service users positive feedback can include the following:

- increasing carers' expectations of the service user
- giving the service user a positive self-image
- giving the service user more opportunities to thrive.

Having read through the above, you may now see that there is always a reason for behaviour. The question you need to ask when it does occur is 'Why is this happening?'

The service user may by experiencing:

- a toothache

- an infection – perhaps an ear infection or urinary tract infection
- a hypo/hyperglycaemic episode which accompanies diabetes
- hypothyroidism – a reduced level of thyroid hormone, particularly common to people with Down syndrome. When the level is low it can cause many problems e.g. fatigue, constipation and depression. These in turn can cause the service user to act differently, especially if the service user does not understand what is happening, is in pain, or is tired or depressed and also unable to explain how he or she is feeling
- fear – perhaps a service user with dementia is scared because she cannot remember where her husband is
- premenstrual tension
- boredom
- frustration.

It is unlikely that you will be able to tell what the problem is until you get to know the service user or until the service user has tools available to help him to communicate.

> Remember: a problem for one person is not always a problem for another. One carer may say that a service user is challenging because he is pacing the floor – most shouldn't find this challenging or even an issue.

FEELINGS

Feelings are at the root of challenging behaviour, which can arise from all different kinds of feelings. These often depend on a service user's ability to do things. For example, a person with dementia may keep forgetting things and thus become embarrassed. An older person may not be able to wash themselves any more and needs a carer to do this, but finds the situation humiliating. A person with a learning disability may want to go shopping by herself but does not have the sense of safety she needs to make the journey safely and feels angry because she does not understand why she is prevented from going.

Being unable to do what you want to do upsets all of us and as one of the people the service user sees regularly, you may find that they take out their anger and frustration on you. You need to remember that you must not take it personally, but must be calm and remain professional.

Below, we explore a range of feelings and how they can lead to challenging behaviour.

STRESS

The people you support can feel stressed now and again, as we all do. How they show it will depend on what is causing the stress, the level of stress and how the service user is able to cope with it and express it. Some people can cope with stress well, others cannot.

Examples of things that can cause stress:

- not having a choice or not being involved in decision making
- living with other people who shout or have the radio or TV on really loud
- finding dirty dishes left in the sink

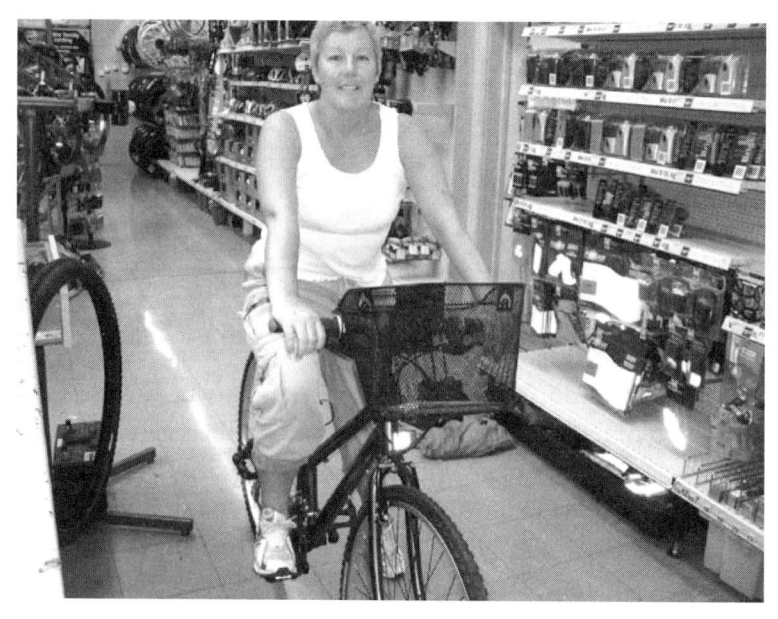

Exercising can help to alleviate stress

- having arguments on what to have for tea or what to watch on TV.

Whatever the disagreement, you will need to try to resolve it and you can do this by:

- talking in a firm, calm voice
- listening to both sides
- reaching a compromise.

> Exercising can alleviate stress and you don't have to go to the gym: walking, swimming and riding a bicycle are just some examples of good forms of exercise.

FEAR AND ANXIETY

> Flight = Running away
> Fight = Staying and fighting

When we are unsure about something or something frightens us, the instinct of 'fight or flight' comes in to play: we have a choice of running away (flight) or staying and facing it (fight).

These reactions are common to all of us, and most times people choose to walk or run away from the thing that is frightening. This can be done quietly by saying, 'I do not like this, I need to go' before leaving or it can be done more demonstratively, by running away fast. Many service users can say 'I don't like this, I need to go.' However, many are unable to communicate in this way, and may take flight by demonstrating behaviour that is challenging, such as throwing things, pushing people etc.

Knowing what can cause a service user to be upset and anxious is one way of trying to prevent it happening.

These 'causes' are called 'trigger points'. Here are some examples of what or who can cause anxieties which can lead to trigger points. On pp.47–54, this list is repeated, but with examples of what to do to prevent these trigger points.

THE ENVIRONMENT

> While its causes include biological factors, it is becoming increasingly clear that it is partly a consequence of the organization of service environments and the behaviour of staff working in those environments. (Department of Health 2001)

CHECKLISTS: ACTIONS AND SITUATIONS THAT CAN LEAD TO CHALLENGING BEHAVIOUR

Environmental issues that can affect behaviour

✎ Please tick the situations that you have seen in your workplace which could contribute to challenging behaviour.

Environmental issue	✓
Service users being prevented from personalizing their own rooms with photos, their own colour scheme and so on	
Rooms are too hot or too cold, but service users are prevented from touching the heating controls; instead, they have to wait for a timer to switch it off	
Dark, unstimulating and/or gloomy environment, which can cause a service user to feel unhappy	
A messy or dirty living space, which can make the service user feel unvalued	
Problems with control of the TV or radio – for example, if a service user would like to watch a wildlife programme on TV but a soap opera is on, or if the radio is on too loud and he cannot get up to adjust the volume	
Irritating noises, such as the dripping of a tap in a service user's bedroom	
Loud colours and bold patterns, which may affect those with sensory issues, or who are struggling with a headache	
Furniture being moved around without consultation	
Lack of privacy – it can be frustrating if there is nowhere to hold a conversation in private	
Curtains being closed by staff without asking	
Service user is angry as he is always left to do the washing up	
Service user was hoping that his favourite member of staff would be on duty to help him	
Service user has been out all day, perhaps in the town drinking, or at college or day centre, and comes back to the home in a lively mood and starts ordering other service users about	

Staff actions that can affect behaviour

✎ Please tick those that are relevant to your workplace.

Staff action	✓
Talking among themselves and excluding service users from conversations	
Talking loudly or not communicating clearly so the service user cannot understand	
Writing in service users' diaries or support plans in front of them without informing the service users what the staff member is writing. Service users may think staff are writing something negative	
Visiting a service user's home but not having time to stay for a chat	
Using closed body language – folded arms, continual staring, pointing, hands on hips – giving the impression that the staff member is angry or disappointed	
Failing to communicate with service users using their preferred form of communication	
Not listening to service users, asking their opinion or following their support plans	
Insisting that the service user does something 'now' rather than in the service user's own time	
Failing to acknowledge cultural or religious beliefs, for example by failing to acknowledge fasting times. Not acknowledging different cultures is very disrespectful	
Insisting that the service user should bathe rather than have a shower, even if showering is their preference	
Failing to dress appropriately, for example, a female member of staff wearing a very short skirt	
Wearing strong perfume or aftershave, which can be overpowering, and also may remind a service user of something or someone from the past	
Individual members of staff being inconsistent and treating different service users differently	
Different members of staff behaving inconsistently: for example, if a service user is learning to make a cup of tea, one staff member teaches him to pour the milk in the cup first, another to put the tea in the cup first	
Using an angry tone of voice or shouting at service users	
Forcing instead of encouraging service users to do a task	
Saying 'No' or giving instructions without explaining why	
Having a negative attitude towards the people that staff support or colleagues	
Having arguments between members of staff, which can upset service users	
Arriving ten minutes late at a service user's home to do personal care	
Displaying behaviours or habits which can cause irritation or offence, for example clicking the lid of a pen repeatedly	

Service users' experiences that can affect behaviour

✎ Please tick those that are relevant to your workplace

Service users' experience	✓
Finding it difficult to communicate: for example, when a service user would like to stop taking sugar in his tea but cannot tell staff as he has no way of communicating it	
Changes to a service user's capability to communicate can be frustrating – for example, experiencing difficulties in communication following a stroke	
Needing comfort – perhaps someone to give a cuddle or hug	
The service user cannot hear properly and wants to ask the staff a question but is nervous as the hearing aid is not working adequately	
Suffering with poor health – e.g. constipation, arthritis	
Tiredness	
Lack of tiredness – inactivity during the day may lead to wandering during the night	
Feeling anxious and untrusting when among new staff	
Experiencing poor care	
Death of a family member, friend, staff or anyone that the service user knows, or other service users talking about their bereavement	
Disturbed sleep – another service user playing their music until late into the night. The service user may worry about the consequences of making a complaint, or may not be able to do so	
Feeling insecure due to changes in routine	
Feeling that personal space has been invaded (particularly common in service users on the autism spectrum)	
Disturbed by the noise from mobile phone texts or calls	
Simply having a bad day at the home, day centre or college	
Boredom – often expressed by pacing the floor	
The service user likes to wear blue all the time and staff say he should wear different colours	
Experiencing side-effects of medication	
Being in an unfamiliar surroundings, e.g. if the service user does not know where he is it can cause him to feel unsafe	
Being scared of perceived dangers – for example shadows cast from trees outside in the bedroom at night	
The service user is a female muslim and will only speak to female muslim GPs. A female muslim GP is not available andf the service user gets distressed and angry	

CAUSES OF CHALLENGING BEHAVIOUR

The weather is sunny and the service user wants to go out or it is raining and the service user has nothing to distract him so it is a gloomy and depressing day
A service user who is an older person does not like to be supported with personal care by a very young carer
A service user has sexual feelings and would like to be intimate. Remember, there is no upper age limit to having sexual feelings and wanting to be intimate and this can include older people with dementia
Tea is being cooked, pots and pans are on the cooker boiling and you ask a service user to put his cup in the kitchen. Depending on the service user's understanding he may be able to do this, he may not. With activities happening in the kitchen, the service user could get confused or upset over what is being asked of him, as the service user may think that you are asking for him to help cook the tea.
Lack of staff time, e.g. the service user needs reassurance from staff but staff are too busy for the service user to ask them a question
Being supported by so many different staff and some not introducing themselves
Dislikes the approach of the staff member
Lack of privacy
Consistent hearing of the buzzing of the call bell, especially during the night
The time of the year e.g. Christmas can be an emotional time, not only financially but also not seeing relatives etc. Winter can be a very depressing time especially if the service user suffers from Seasonal Affective Disorder (SAD).
Other service users' challenging behaviour

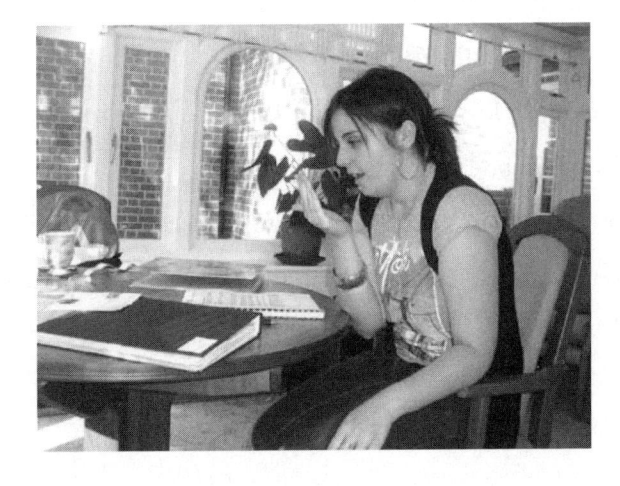

Tiredness can cause challenging behaviour

Parents' and relatives' actions that can affect behaviour

✎ Please tick those that are relevant to your workplace.

Parents' and relatives' action	✓
Treating the service user who is an adult like a child, by not giving them choices or talking over their head	
Not enabling the service user to do things for himself; always doing things for him, even when done with good intentions	
Talking about the service user in his presence in a way that embarrasses him	
Not respecting the service user's choices – for example, demanding that he wear a tracksuit when he has chosen a smart shirt and trousers to wear	

✎ Can you think of any more? List them here:

....
....
....
....

LOSS AND CHANGE

Experiences of loss and change are a common cause of anxiety and challenging behaviour. Types of loss can range from bereavement through to the loss of familiar routines or habits. They can include:

- loss of family members
- loss of a pet or animal
- staff leaving – loss of the person, and also their routines
- loss of independence
- loss of physical or mental capabilities, perhaps due to illness.

The need to support service users through their loss or change is not always recognized by staff who work closely with the service users.

✎ Are the people you care for given help and support when:

- a person or an animal has died? Yes/No

CAUSES OF CHALLENGING BEHAVIOUR

- a member of staff is due to leave or has already left, perhaps did not return from sick leave?   Yes/No

- a new staff member starts?   Yes/No

- coming to terms with the loss of independence due to illness or an accident?   Yes/No

- someone arrives at a residential home having lived independently for years?   Yes/No

✒ If you have answered 'No' to any of these, please complete the chart on what you think the consequences are for the service user and what you can do about it

The loss or change	What are the consequences to the service user if support is not offered?	What can you do about it?
A much-loved pet has died		
A member of staff does not return from sick leave		
A new staff member starts working in their place		
A older service user with dementia has lived independently with his wife for many years, but yesterday moved into a residential home		
Coming to terms with the loss of independence due to illness or an accident		

Reacting and Responding to Challenging Behaviour

How you react to challenging behaviour can make a big difference to how the person exhibiting the behaviour feels, and also whether they continue with the behaviour.

FEELINGS AND REACTIONS

Whether you are a service user or staff, remembering your feelings and reactions prior to, during and after a challenging incident can be different for each person. Some feel very anxious; others feel quite relaxed and become stressed only after an event.

What we all have in common is:

The adrenaline flows and the liver releases glucose
to help muscles work effectively
↓
Breathing gets faster which results in an increase in blood pressure
↓
Churning stomach and dry mouth can happen
as blood is diverted from the digestive system
↓
Muscles tense
↓
Pupils widen to help us see clearer

Once an incident has finished the body should return to normal.

If the incident has a long duration your body will continue to do the above; in turn, this could be unhealthy, and this is what leads to stress.

WHAT SHOULD YOU DO WHEN SOMEONE PRESENTS CHALLENGING BEHAVIOUR?

Support in a non-confrontational planned way and follow guidance. Do not stand directly in front of the service user. When people are upset and angry they can go through various stages of emotions and behaviours, and this is called the Five Stages of Emotional Arousal: triggering, build-up, crisis, recovery and post-crisis depression.

1. *Triggering*: challenging behaviour is always caused by something and this is called a 'trigger'. There can be various triggers and you will have read some examples of these on previous pages.

    What should I do?
    - You need to monitor what is happening and inform others.
    - Try to divert the service user's attention to something he likes, or provide the opportunity for the service user to have some quiet time away from others if he wishes.

2. *Build-up*: you will notice changes in the person. The service user may become more agitated, or more active, become abusive and breathe heavily. In advanced stages the service user may be unpredictable and you will need to think about what you do, what you say and how you approach the service user.

    What should I do?
    - Approach in a careful manner.
    - Have an open body language, with fists open so the service user can see you do not have anything in your hands and with your shoulders relaxed.
    - Try to understand the reasons why the service user is doing what he is doing.
    - Respond and listen to what the service user is telling you.

3. *Crisis*: if it gets to the crisis stage, this means that the service user has lost control and can be aggressive and/or violent.

What should I do?

- Do what the support plan, risk assessment or behavioural guidelines tell you to do; e.g. if it says things like: 'Do not approach', 'Do not get too close', 'Do not have your back to the service user or to a door' or 'Do not corner the service user as this could make him scared', then *do not do it!*

- Observe regularly: how this should be done and how often will depend on the service user.

- Be safe: if the support plan, risk assessment or behavioural guidelines say that you should go to people's homes in twos or walk around the residential setting in twos to safeguard yourselves, then you must do this, and call for back-up if needed.

- Look at ways to defuse the situation, perhaps by diverting the attention of the service user to something that he likes if it is safe to do so.

- Maintain normal eye contact (blink occasionally, do not stare). This shows concern for the service user, reinforcing that you are there for support and that you are not apprehensive.

- Use peripheral vision: vision from the corner of your eye. This will enable you to see what is happening with the service user's hands and feet, see who else is entering the room and check whether anyone else is in distress.

- Keep your voice at a low level and calm tone; this shows concern rather than agitation, reinforcing that you are in control of the situation, preventing you from showing signs of agitation or apprehension.

- Try to understand why the person is anxious.

- Respond in a way that shows you are listening.

- Do not make promises that you may not be able to complete.

- Keep your facial expression neutral: this prevents you showing any negative feelings and prevents your eye contact becoming a stare.

- Remember that if the service user is still anxious, it may reach the crisis stage, e.g. the service user has become irrational and possibly lost control: you need to be thinking about yourself and others in the area.
- Try to reassure the service user and follow any behavioural programmes or risk assessments that are written to support the service user.
- Keep your hands at waist height in a non-confrontational way, open to gestures and providing protection, i.e. you can use your arms to block any blows that may come your way.
- Stand sideways on: this is non-confrontational and means you can move quickly from the area if needed.

4. *Recovery*: when the service user is beginning to relax, we call this 'recovery'. Some may recover quickly, others may take a lot longer.

What should I do?

- Offer reassurance.
- Avoid the trigger that started the situation and any other triggers.
- Offer activities or opportunities that will change the person's frame of mind and make him feel better.

5. *Post-crisis depression*: some service users may become withdrawn or feel low after an incident and may find it difficult to talk.

What should I do?

- Follow the written guidance as this will tell you if the service user would like to be left alone, or offered support and activities that will help him to feel better.
- Understand that the service user may like counselling: this can be an informal conversation with yourself or you could arrange for professional counselling.

WHAT TO DO AFTER THE INCIDENT

Your policies and procedures will tell you what you should do after an incident and may include completing a chart to record what happened before, during and after the incident. This is called an ABC chart and an example of this can be found on p.88.

✍ Ask your manager what you should do if you are at risk and write your answers here:

If I am at risk I should:

....
....
....

TOUCH

As care staff you can use physical guidance, i.e. place your hand over the hand of the service user to support them when carrying out activities they may find difficult, such as pouring juice, using a vacuum cleaner or polishing surfaces. Doing so acts as a prompt, to help the service user to learn a skill. However, if a service user resists for more than a few seconds, this is no longer teaching: the service user is telling you that he does not want to do the task and does not want you to touch him. Therefore, you must stop the activity immediately and inform your manager.

Some organizations have a blanket policy that there should be no touching between staff and service users, which includes hugging, etc. Others have a policy that says, if the hug is instigated by the service user, then this is OK.

✍ Look at your organization's policy. What does it say about touch? Write your answer here:

....
....
....

PHYSICAL INTERVENTION AND RESTRAINT

Below is a brief definition of restraint:

> The use or threat of force to help do an act which the person resists, or the restriction of the person's liberty of movement, whether or not they resist. Restraint may only be used where it is necessary to protect the person from

harm and is proportionate to the risk of harm. (Mental Capacity Act 2005 Code of Practice Section 6[4])

The Care Quality Commission's guidance on restraint says:

> Restraint is illegal unless it can be demonstrated that for an individual in particular circumstances not being restrained would conflict with the duty of care of the service. And that the outcome for the individual would be harm to themselves or for others.
>
> Where people in care services have capacity restraint may only take place with their consent or in an emergency to prevent harm to themselves or others or to prevent a crime being committed. (Care Quality Commission 2009)

More information can be obtained from the CQC website: www.cqc.org.uk/guidanceforprofessionals/socialcare/careproviders/guidance.cfm

Some service users may be on a physical intervention programme for a period of time, which means that during this period staff can physically intervene if the service user is at risk or putting others at risk.

This programme must be agreed by the multidisciplinary team and your manager will put you on a training course to learn the intervention techniques that you can use with that particular service user. You will also learn how and when to use it and how and when to complete the physical intervention book.

Guidance on restraint policy

> The policies and practices of the home ensure that physical and/or verbal aggression by service users is understood and dealt with appropriately, and that physical intervention is used only as a last resort and in accordance with DH guidance. (Department of Health 2000b)

> The misuse of physical restraint has resulted in many injuries, and in the most serious case, deaths. If restraint is seen to be necessary to maintain an individual's safety, or the safety of others, the agreed methods of how and when it should be used must be clearly detailed, and those involved in the intervention must have received the appropriate training. (CQC 2009)

PHYSICAL INTERVENTION

> The policies and practices of the home ensure that physical and/or verbal aggression by service users is understood and dealt with appropriately, and that

physical intervention is used only as a last resort and in accordance with DH guidance. (CQC Care Home for Older People Standard 18.5)

Physical and verbal aggression by a service user is understood and dealt with appropriately, and physical intervention is used only as a last resort by trained staff in accordance with Department of Health guidance, protects the rights and best interests of the service user, and is the minimum consistent with safety. (CQC Care Home for Adults Standard 23.5)

Physical and verbal aggression by a service user, their relatives or friends is responded to appropriately. Physical intervention is only used as a last resort, in accordance with Department of Health guidance and protects the rights and best interests of the service user, including people with special needs and is the minimum necessary consistent with safety. (CQC Domiciliary Standard 14.6)

WHAT *NOT* TO DO WHEN RESPONDING TO CHALLENGING BEHAVIOUR

When responding to challenging behaviour, you must *not* do any of the following:

- Withhold food, drink, medication, clothes or bedding.
- Use medication to control the behaviour unless agreed by the doctor and the multidisciplinary team. This is known as chemical restraint or covert medication.
- Withhold services such as access to doctors, dentists, hospital appointments etc.
- Tie service users to furniture or fixtures.
- Prevent the service user from moving – whether by putting the cot sides up or tucking blankets in so tightly that the service user cannot move or positioning a table so the service user cannot move.
- Use seclusion or time out. If a service user is upset and chooses to go to his room to 'chill out', he *must be allowed* to close the door; staff must not close the door on him.
- Use any technique that could cause physical pain or injury, i.e. holds that 'lock' joints.
- Lock doors.

- Use threats.
- Remove hearing aid, glasses or walking aids.
- Keep service user in his nightwear so he cannot go out or leave his room.
- Use surveillance to monitor and/or restrict people's actions and movements, including the use of electronic surveillance, pressure pads by doors or electronic tags.
- Make a service user scared of doing what he wants to do and making him think that he has no other option, e.g. stay living where he is.

✎ Can you think of any more?

....
....
....
....

What should I do if I witness any of the above happening?

There are several things you can do:

- Discuss your concerns with your manager.
- If it is abuse and your manager is not doing anything about it, you should go to your manager's manager.
- If there is not another manager for you to go to, you should make a safeguarding referral to social services.

The workbook *Safeguarding Adults*, also in this series, will give you more information on what abuse is, how to prevent it happening and what to do if it is happening.

> Remember: it is everyone's duty to protect vulnerable children and adults.

Self-Harm

Self-harm is a form of challenging behaviour which you may or may not encounter in your workplace, but it is useful for you to understand what it is and why people can choose to do it.

> The term 'self-harm' includes many behaviours, including cutting, burning, scalding, banging, or scratching your own body; breaking bones; pulling hair; and ingesting toxic substances or objects. The practice is often dismissed as a cry for help, a primitive method of attention seeking. However, […] most cases of self-harm are hidden, particularly from friends and family.
>
> Chris Holley stated at a Royal College of Nursing conference in April 2006, 'It's about people who self injure in order to manage their feelings and live rather than die.' These coping strategies give a temporary fix for people who see no other way of managing emotional distress. For many people self-harm is a private activity that they do not want to discuss with anyone. (Kinmond and Kinmond 2006)

✎ What are your views on these two paragraphs?

....
....
....
....

✎ Complete the following with your supervisor. To promote service users' rights to confidentiality, please do not write their names.

Have you had any experience of supporting people
who self-harm?   Yes / No

Picking one individual, what is your opinion of the fact that they self-harm?

....
....
....
....

SELF-HARM

Are there guidelines in your workplace to support the service
user when he or she self-harms? Yes/No

What do you know about the guidelines?

．．．
．．．
．．．
．．．

How has the service user self-harmed?

．．．
．．．
．．．
．．．

Why do you think the service user self-harms?

．．．
．．．
．．．
．．．

What can you do to help?

．．．
．．．
．．．
．．．

How could you make it worse?

．．．
．．．
．．．
．．．

What do you think are the benefits to the service user who self-harms?

....
....
....
....

What effect does a person self-harming have on the people they live with: family, friends and the staff team?

....
....
....
....

SERVICE USERS SECTIONED OR DETAINED AGAINST THEIR WILL

The Mental Health Act 1983 as amended by the Mental Health Act 2007 gives powers to detain people in hospital for assessment and treatment (see Department of Health 2008).

Some people who are defined as having severe challenging behaviour, mental illness, psychopathic disorder, severe mental impairment, for example, may place themselves or others in danger and therefore may be sectioned or detained against their will under the Mental Health Act 1983 as a formal patient.

Informal patients:

The vast majority of the people receiving treatment in a mental hospital* or psychiatric unit are **informal patients**, which means they are in hospital on a voluntary basis and have exactly the same rights as a person being treated for a physical illness.

Formal patients, who constitute about 20 per cent of the mental hospital population, are *compulsorily* detained under a section of the Mental Health Act 1983 and lose some of the rights available to informal patients. (Department of Health 2008)

For more information go to www.mind.org.uk/help/rights_and_legislation/mental_health_act_1983_an_outline_guide

---

*   Mental hospital is an old term for a psychiatric hospital.

How to Minimize and/or Prevent Challenging Behaviour

Each display of behaviour and the reason behind it is unique to the individual service user and the strategies below have been tried and tested by me when I have supported people with learning disabilities and challenging behaviour.

Many years ago I asked someone in the care profession why one of her staff shouted at the service users. She said that the worker was often told not to shout, and that in doing so she was probably:

- causing upset to the service user
- showing she was nervous
- shouting at the service user so she could be in control because she did not have any control in her own life.

You must not shout at service users at any time. This includes when the service user is challenging. You should speak firmly when you need to but do not shout.

WAYS OF WORKING TO PROMOTE POSITIVE RELATIONSHIPS AND REDUCE CHALLENGING BEHAVIOUR

When I have been asked by managers to do some training with their staff on challenging behaviour, I always arrange to go into the service a few evenings beforehand and observe what is actually happening, so my observations can form part of the training.

When I arrive, some staff may say about a service user, 'He's attention seeking', and I explain that we all need some attention and some service users cannot do the things they would like to do, or occupy themselves without support. I then ask them what interaction and support the service user is getting from staff. The answers often cover the basics, e.g. 'He is supported to get washed and dressed, eat his meals and go to the day centre.'

During the training session that follows, staff receive knowledge on how to support the service user in a person-centred way, for example:

- seeing the service user as a person
- seeing the service user as someone with rights, needs and wishes
- seeing the service user first and the behaviour second
- paying attention to positive behaviour and where possible ignoring negative behaviour
- not making judgements on why the service user is displaying a particular behaviour
- providing an active structured day for the service user
- providing a consistent response to challenging behaviour.

When we are worried and/or distressed, our anxiety levels increase and we need reassurance more so than at other times. You may have experienced this with a person with a learning disability or an older person who has dementia.

Spending time with a service user on a one-to-one basis, either involved in a conversation or sometimes just listening to the service user, or even just giving eye contact and a smile, can mean a lot to the individual service user.

Praise the service user for things he does well and ignore behaviour which could be perceived as challenging if there is no risk involved. If he presents challenging behaviour, gently divert his attention to something he enjoys doing.

You will now read on the next pages causes or triggers of behaviour and on the right hand side what can be done to prevent the behaviour.

Environmental issues

✍ Please tick those behaviours that you have observed in your workplace.

Cause	✓	Reduce
Service users being prevented from personalizing their own rooms with photos, their own colour scheme, and so on		Service users should be encouraged to personalize their own rooms with photos and their own colour scheme as this shows their individuality and identity.

HOW TO MINIMIZE AND/OR PREVENT CHALLENGING BEHAVIOUR

Rooms are too hot or too cold, but service users are prevented from touching heating controls; instead, they have to wait for a timer to switch off	The heating will probably be on a timer, however, staff need to be aware that rooms can cool during the day and if the service users are not active they will feel the cold and need to be encouraged to wear clothing appropriate for the weather. You could discuss this individually with your manager ort raise it at a staff meeting.
Dark, unstimulating and/or gloomy environment, which can cause a service user to feel unhappy	Introduce a bright, warm environment, free of clutter.
A messy or dirty living space, which can make the service user feel unvalued	Sometimes areas can get like this if the service user is depressed. You could encourage the service user to clean it or offer a helping hand and do it together.
Problems with control of the TV or radio – for example, if a service user would like to watch a wildlife programme on TV but a soap opera is on, or if the radio is on too loud and he cannot get up to adjust the volume	At the beginning of the week you could sit with the service user and go through the TV magazine and outline what the service user would like to watch.
Irritating noises, such as the dripping of a tap in a service user's bedroom	You need to report this immediately and if possible, put something in the sink which can cushion the noise of the water hitting the sink, e.g. a cup or flannel.
Loud colours and bold patterns, which may affect those with sensory issues, or who are struggling with a headache	You can discuss this with the service user and the manager; perhaps the colours and patterns can be toned done a little. If the service user has a headache encourage him/her to go to a quieter area.
Furniture being moved around without consultation	Discuss any changes with the service user and where possible do the changes with the service user.
Lack of privacy – it can be frustrating if there is nowhere to hold a conversation in private	There will be other room(s)/areas available within the home where service users can go for privacy, e.g. the dining room. A bedroom is sometimes used for this but if e.g. you had a meeting with your social worker would you like him/her to be in your bedroom? The people you support may need reminding that they can go to a quieter area/room to talk to their family and friends or staff members or each other
Curtains being closed by staff without asking	Encourage service user to be responsible for closing the curtains.

47

Service user is angry as he is always left to do the washing up		Have regular house meetings where everyone can view their opinions.
Service user was hoping that his favourite member of staff would be on duty to help him		Give the service user a copy of the rota (use photographs if needed). You will need to ensure that the service user will use the rota in the proper way. Some service users like to know when staff are on duty so they can target the staff member.
Service user has been out all day, perhaps in the town drinking, or at college or day centre, and comes back to the home in a lively mood and starts ordering other service users about		It is important that this is stopped before it escalates. Ask the service user to go and do something, e.g. get the washing off the line, anything to divert his attention and get him away from others. While doing the task he is adjusting and calming down. Do this every time he comes back so that he learns what he should do. It is also important in a place where service users are likely to challenge that the service users come home to a peaceful house, no blaring music or numerous radios with different stations. A peaceful home will have a calming affect on the service users.

Staff actions

✍ Please tick those that are relevant to your workplace.

Cause	✓	Reduce
Talking among themselves and excluding service users from conversations		If talking privately, do it away from the service users; if you are talking about what you did last night, save it until you finish duty.
Talking loudly or not communicating clearly so the service user cannot understand		You should keep your voice at your normal pace, pitch and conversational level. If you are stressed or anxious do some deep breathing and count to ten.
Writing in service users' diaries or support plans in front of them without informing the service users what the staff member is writing. Service users may think staff are writing something negative		Explain to the service user what you are going to write and why you need to write it.

Visiting a service user's home but not having time to stay for a chat	You may have allocated time to provide care and support, and while doing this you should be talking with the service user. If the service user wants more time to chat, inform him/her you will discuss it with the manager.
Using closed body language – folded arms, continual staring, pointing, hands on hips – giving the impression that the staff member is angry or disappointed	You can cause or escalate anxiety by your body language. Keep your body language open.
Failing to communicate with service users using their preferred form of communication	Use the service user's preferred method of communication. If needed devise photos etc. with the service user.
Not listening to service users, asking their opinion or following their support plans	It is disrespectful to do this and it can confuse the service user if you are not following the support plan.
Insisting that the service user does something 'now' rather than in the service user's own time	Inform the service user what needs to be done, why it needs to be done and ask when the time would be convenient to do it.
Failing to acknowledge cultural or religious beliefs, for example by failing to acknowledge fasting times	Keep a calendar and write on it religious festivals and observations
Insisting that the service user should bathe rather than have a shower, even if showering is their preference	Provide the opportunity for the service user to choose.
Failing to dress appropriately, for example, a female member of staff wearing a very short skirt	You must dress appropriately: wear clothes that are loose enough to move about but that are not revealing or skirts that are too short. You should avoid slogans on clothes which may cause offence.
Wearing a strong perfume or aftershave, which can be overpowering and also may remind a service user of something or someone from the past	Avoid using strong perfumes and be aware that smells can create physical and emotional reactions.
Individual members of staff being inconsistent and treating different service users differently	Take care to treat all service users equally and with respect.

Different members of staff behaving inconsistently: for example, if a service user is learning to make a cup of tea, one staff member teaches him to pour the milk in the cup first, another to put the tea in the cup first	Write a step-by-step programme on how the service user will be supported to make a cup of tea and all staff will follow the same approach.
Using an angry tone of voice or shouting at service users	You should use an even tone of voice; if the guidelines say you need to be firm verbally then be firm, but do not shout or get angry.
Forcing instead of encouraging service users to do a task	You should encourage and if needed offer an incentive.
Saying 'No' or giving instructions without explaining why	Always explain why something cannot happen and back it up when it can happen.
Having a negative attitude towards the people that staff support or colleagues	If you go to work in a bad mood it can have a knock-on effect on the people you support and work with. Leave your problems at the front door.
Having arguments between members of staff, which can upset service users	If you have any problems with staff you should discuss them in your supervision meeting with your manager or supervisor. If your supervision isn't for a while, ask your manager if you can have a quick word and tell him/her and get it sorted.
Arriving ten minutes late at a service user's home to do personal care	Ten minutes may not seem a lot to you but if a service user's support is due to arrive at 11am to give a bath, the service user has already been waiting a long time. Apologize to the service user and ensure it does not happen again. Do not then go on and on about it, simply apologize and then concentrate on what the service user wants. In future, be aware of the time and be punctual.
Displaying behaviours or habits which can cause irritation or offence, for example clicking the lid of a pen repeatedly	This can be very annoying and staff do not always realize they are doing it. Be aware of the habits you have and put yourself in the shoes of the service user.

Service users' experiences

✎ Please tick those that are relevant to your workplace

Cause	✓	Reduce
Finding it difficult to communicate: for example, when a service user would like to stop taking sugar in his tea but cannot tell staff as he has no way of communicating it		Needs change regularly and the service user could be asked each time how he would like his tea by asking one question at a time.
Changes to a service user's capability to communicate can be frustrating – for example, experiencing difficulties in communication following a stroke		You could put together a small album of photos that the service user can point to as a way of saying what he wants.
Needing comfort – perhaps someone to give a cuddle or hug		This will depend on your policy and procedure on touch. You could also look into helping the service user to build friendship or social networks.
The service user cannot hear properly and wants to ask the staff a question but is nervous as the hearing aid is not working adequately		The hearing aid should be checked regularly. The relationship between staff and service users should not be a strained one.
Suffering with poor health – e.g. constipation, arthritis		Observe the service user. Has he got the skills or tools to communicate and tell you what is wrong?
Tiredness		Observe the service user and you will see when he/she is tired.
Lack of tiredness – inactivity during the day may lead to wandering during the night		Encourage the service user to do some activities during the day, even if it is just a few walks around the garden.
Feeling anxious and untrusting when among new staff		Provide opportunities for the new staff to meet and get to know the service user.
Experiencing poor care		Poor care should be reported to the manager.
Death of a family member, friend, staff or anyone that the service user knows, or other service users talking about their bereavement		It is important that the staff acknowledge that service users need to grieve the same as everyone else. The service users need time to acknowledge and talk through what has happened. This can be with someone of his choice e.g. family, a staff member, a counsellor etc.
Disturbed sleep – another service user playing their music until late into the night. The service user may worry about the consequences of making a complaint, or may not be able to do so		Ensure the service user knows how to complain. If the music is loud you will hear it too. You can then ask the other service user to turn it down.

Feeling insecure due to changes in routine	Give advance warnings of any changes and the reasons for these changes.
Feeling that personal space has been invaded (particularly common in service users on the autism spectrum)	Don't stand too close to the service user.
Disturbed by the noise from mobile phone texts or calls	Most organizations tell staff that they should not have their mobile phones turned on while at work.
Simply having a bad day at the home, day centre or college	Provide an opportunity to discuss this with the service user and ask if there is anything that can be done to make it better.
Boredom – often expressed by pacing the floor	Provide an opportunity to discuss things he may like to do. Sometimes you may need to suggest options for the service user.
The service user likes to wear blue all the time and staff say he should wear different colours	If the service user chooses to wear blue all the time, you could suggest to him that he wears different shades of blue perhaps.
Experiencing side-effects of medication	Read up on the side-effects and consult the GP.
Being in unfamiliar surroundings, e.g. if the service user does not know where he is it can cause him to feel unsafe	When trying a new activity or going to a new place, you can take photos and show the service user, or look it up on the Internet, or if it is going to the cinema for the first time why not go there and look at it from the outside and then discuss how the service user feels. Next time go in and see if he feels comfortable. If not, come back and next time go in and watch the film.
Being scared of percieved dangers – for example shadows cast from trees outside in the bedroom at night	You can reassure the service user that it is the tree, arrange for the branches to be trimmed or ask the service user if he would like blacked out curtains.
The service user is a female Muslim and will only speak to female Muslim GPs. A female Muslim GP is not available and the service user gets distressed and angry.	When making an appointment explain the service user's preference to see a female Muslim GP.
The weather is sunny and the service user wants to go out or it is raining and the service user has nothing to distract him so it is a gloomy and depressing day	Acknowledge the reason and suggest other things to do.
A service user who is an older person does not like to be supported with personal care by a very young carer	This would need to be discussed with the manager.

A service user has sexual feelings and would like to be intimate. Remember, there is no upper age limit to having sexual feelings and wanting to be intimate and this can include older people with dementia	This would need to be discussed with the manager.
Tea is being cooked, pots and pans are on the cooker boiling and you ask a service user to put his cup in the kitchen. Depending on the service user's understanding he may be able to do this, he may not. With activities happening in the kitchen, the service user could get confused or upset over what is being asked of him, as the service user may think that you are asking for him to help cook the tea.	You could choose a different time to ask the service user to put the cup in the kitchen.
Lack of staff time, e.g. the service user needs reassurance from staff but staff are too busy for the service user to ask them a question	This could be discussed with the manager.
Being supported by so many different staff and some not introducing themselves	This could be discussed with the manager.
Dislikes the approach of the staff member	This could be discussed with the manager and brought up in the staff member's supervision.
Lack of privacy	It is important that privacy is respected at all times.
Consistent hearing of the buzzing of the call bell, especially during the night	This needs to be discussed with the manager: perhaps a different system could be in place where it beeps to a gadget that the carer has in her pocket.
The time of the year e.g. Christmas can be an emotional time, not only financially but also not seeing relatives etc. Winter can be a very depressing time especially if the service user suffers from Seasonal Affective Disorder (SAD).	Before winter arrives start planning with the service user and the team what you can do to reduce these emotional periods.
Other service users' challenging behaviour	Ensure you follow the guidelines for the service users who are challenging which will no doubt include something about protecting the other service users.

A service user approaches and shouts at another service user and a fight starts. You take the side of the service user who shouted and this makes the service user who was shouted at very angry	You should discuss the unacceptable behaviour with both service users, starting with the service user who started it by shouting.
The unknown, e.g. the service user and the staff member are about to do something together and the staff leaves the service user waiting while the staff does something else	Before asking a service user to do something with you, make sure you have done everything you need to do so you will not be distracted.

Parents' and relatives' actions

✎ Please tick those that are relevant to your workplace.

Cause	✓	Reduce
Treating the service user who is an adult like a child, by not giving them choices or talking over their head		Show respect at all times.
Not enabling the service user to do things for himself; always doing things for him, even when done with good intentions		Encourage the service user to do things for himself, such as invite his mum for a coffee and support service user to make it.
Talking about the service user in his presence in a way that embarrasses him		Show respect at all times.
Not respecting the service user's choices – for example demanding that he wear a tracksuit when he has chosen a smart shirt and trousers to wear		Explain that the service user should be encouraged to make choices. You should also explain the service user's rights to the parents but make sure you do it in a sensitive way. Remember that no matter what age people are, parents usually want a say in a person's life.

STRATEGIES FOR MINIMIZING CHALLENGING BEHAVIOUR: USING POSITIVE REINFORCEMENTS

- Build a professional relationship with the people you support so they can tell you when they are feeling upset or angry.
- You may then be able to prevent something happening.
- Discuss what is upsetting the service user and suggest ways of reducing the upset.

We all need to be praised for doing things well, e.g. 'Well done, you did that brilliantly,' or being made a cup of tea or taken out for a meal to celebrate an achievement etc. Each time we are praised it raises our self-esteem and it makes us feel good so that we want to do well again to get that praise. We then continue to do well to get the praise and feel good.

We all like to hear people say 'Thank you' when we have done something for them.

✍ Do you say 'Thank you' when a service user has done something that you have asked him to do?   Yes/No

Explain why:

....
....
....
....

> If we never get recognized for the things we do well, it could be that we are recognized only for the things we do badly. This is negative and if we get recognized only for doing things badly, we may continue to do things badly so we get the attention and get recognized.

STRATEGIES FOR MINIMIZING CHALLENGING BEHAVIOUR: SUPPORT PLANS AND CARE PLANS

Some organizations have support plans, other organizations call them care plans, but they all fill the same purpose.

> The Plan establishes individualised procedures for service users likely to be aggressive or cause harm or self-harm, focusing on positive behaviour, ability and willingness. (CQC Care Home for Adults Standard 6.5)

✍ What are the plans called in your workplace?

....

For the purpose of this workbook I will refer to these plans as 'support plans' as one of your responsibilities will be to *support* the service user. This means supporting the service user to do things, not taking over and doing things for him, but supporting. When you *support* you *enable* and *empower*.

Working together: job share!

Throughout your time in the care area you will learn that there is great emphasis on *supporting, enabling* and *empowering* service users to do or achieve the things the service user wishes to do or achieve. Sometimes the service user could feel overpowered by always having to do things and perhaps sometimes it is nice to 'job share', e.g. agree with the service user that if he does the washing up you will do the drying or something similar. We all appreciate help sometimes and it is no different for the people you support. But remember, do not take over!

Each service user will have a support plan which will give detailed information on how the individual service user wishes to be supported. This plan will not only cover the basics, i.e. washing, times of getting up etc. but also include more specific tasks that the individual service user wishes to do, and there will be some specific tasks that have goals attached to them that the individual service user wishes to achieve, and details of how the support must be provided and by whom, such as yourself, advocate, social services etc.

You will have read the words *individual service user* quite a bit here and this is because the service user is an individual with his own strengths, needs and wishes. You must not use the same support plan for anyone except for the individual service user it is designed for.

You must ask the service user his preferences. Do not stereotype the people you support by their age, disability, culture, race etc. For example:

- An older person will not necessarily want to watch *Songs of Praise* each Sunday or listen to music by Val Doonican, and he or she may not be deaf.

- Being a person with a learning disability does not automatically mean that he or she will have challenging behaviour.

- A female service user may not always want to wear a dress.

Who builds the plan?

The support plan can be built by many people, e.g.

- the service user

- key worker
- family
- friends
- advocate etc.

Some service users may have two support plans; support plan no. 1 will be when everything is going smoothly and the service user is well, and support plan no. 2 will be used when the service user is not very well – a less well day (in mental health services this is called a crisis plan). Where possible the service user will tell you in advance so it can be recorded on his support plan what he wants you and/or his family to do when he has a 'less well day'.

It is important that you get to know the service user and his/her preferences, needs, wishes and history. All these are very important as they can affect the way the service user may react to situations and here are some examples.

EXAMPLE 1: PREFERENCES

The service user wants to hang his washing on the line with the waist of the trousers pegged on the line. When you do your washing in your home you peg the ends of the legs on the line. It is the service user's preference to put the waist of the trousers on the line and you must not change this. The end result will be the same, i.e. the trousers will dry on the line.

EXAMPLE 2: HISTORY

A service user does not like having his hair washed by staff while in the bath. The staff member told the service user that she was going to wash his hair now but he did not understand what she meant. The water ran into his eyes, he was frightened and got distressed, his first reaction was to push the staff member out of the way. Unfortunately she hit the wall and fell onto the floor. It was not the service user's fault: he did not understand what the staff member said and if she had checked the support plan she would have read that the service user prefers that his hair is washed over the sink.

EXAMPLE 3: NEEDS

A service user with a mental health diagnosis lives by himself in a flat and enjoys living by himself. He receives X number of hours support per week to check his mental well-being and that he is taking his medication on time. You have been visiting for some months now and as he is taking the medication you miss a few visits. During this time the service user has not taken his medication and his mental state has deteriorated; he has become paranoid and thinks that the neighbour is stalking him.

It is important that you are familiar with the support plan, and discuss the plan with your manager if there is anything you do not understand or anything that needs changing. It is important that you yourself do not change or alter the plan without informing others.

Requirements on care planning by the CQC

The plan establishes individualised procedures for service users in relation to the taking of risks in daily living and for those service users who are likely to be aggressive, abusive or cause harm or self-harm, focussing on positive behaviour. (CQC Domiciliary Standards-standard 7)

6.1: The registered manager develops and agrees with each service user a service user Plan, which may include treatment and rehabilitation, describing the services and facilities to be provided by the home, and how these services will meet current and changing needs and aspirations and achieve goals.

6.3: The Plan sets out how current and anticipated specialist requirements will be met [for example through positive planned interventions; rehabilitation and therapeutic programmes; structured environments; development of Language and communication; adaptations and equipment; one-to-one communication support]. (CQC Care Home for Adults Standards)

7.2: The service user's plan sets out in detail the action which needs to be taken by care staff to ensure that all aspects of the health, personal and social care needs of the service user (see Standard 3) are met.

7.4: The service user's plan is reviewed by care staff in the home at least once a month, updated to reflect changing needs and current objectives for health and personal care, and actioned.

7.6: The plan is drawn up with the involvement of the service user, recorded in a style accessible to the service user; agreed and signed.

STRATEGIES FOR MINIMIZING CHALLENGING BEHAVIOUR: STRUCTURING TIME

A structured period of the day for the service user can reduce challenging behaviour. This does not necessarily mean a structured day from the time the service user gets up to the time he goes to bed; some service users need structure for some of the day whereas others may need structure for most of the day or even the whole day!

The structure can enable the people you support to feel relaxed as they know what to expect in their day; not knowing can cause anxieties which can lead to challenging behaviour. Spending quality and meaningful time with the service user can go a long way in you getting to know him/her and vice versa.

It will be difficult for social care workers working in people's homes to provide structures as you are going there for a short period with a specific task to complete. However, if you feel the service user will benefit from a structure, you can discuss this with the manager who will then pass it on to the social worker and/or family.

The people you support will have a care plan or support plan and part of your role as a social care worker may be to check with the service user what he has planned and remind him of certain activities he enjoys which will have previously been identified and written on the care/support plan.

Time

We all have a time when we prefer to do things; whether it is to do the household chores or learn or just when we are more motivated. Is there a 'best time' for the service user to do things, for example does the service user prefer to do things in the morning, afternoon or evening, before or after a cup of tea?

✎ How will you find out the best time to spend time with a service user to get to know him?

....
....

What do you think will happen if you ask a service user to do something and it is not the 'best time' for him?

....
....
....
....

The best time will be when the service user is relaxed, not involved in an activity (unless the service user finds it easier to talk while doing an activity, e.g. potting plants, walking in the park), a time when the service user wants to spend time with you, in an environment or venue that suits you both and one where you can both relax and talk without being interrupted.

If you are meeting the service user for the first time and he cannot speak, you can do the talking and watch his reactions. You will be surprised how much he understands and will respond; this may be in the form of smiling, winking, frowning, shaking a wrist etc.

Before you have this time with the service user, please discuss this with your manager, who will be able to advise you further and if you need to be following any risk assessments or support plans. It is important that you do this as you do not want to put your foot in it and upset the service user by doing or saying the wrong thing.

✎ Do the people you support spend time waiting around doing nothing? Yes/No

If you answered 'Yes' what can you do about this?

....
....
....
....

We all need to be needed and supporting service users to make contributions such as helping with the washing-up, doing some housework, watering the plants or gardening can go a long way in making the service users feel wanted and raise their self-esteem.

If service users are able to occupy themselves then this is OK but if they cannot occupy themselves then the service users could be sitting or standing bored with nothing to do. If this happens then the service users can show through their behaviour how bored they are.

Some people go into residential care for the company but:

- Is the company actually there? Yes/No
- Is the house too noisy so the service user stays in his room? Yes/No
- Does the service user need your help in getting to know the other service users? Yes/No
- Does the service user spend most of his time in his room because he prefers familiar surroundings? Yes/No
- Is the service user frightened to leave his room as staff may go in and clean his room while he is not there? Yes/No
- Is the service user worried that other service users may go in his room? Yes/No

✎ Are the people you support feeling lonely or isolated? Yes/No

If you have answered 'Yes' to the above question, suggest how you can alleviate the loneliness and isolation:

....
....
....
....

Another workbook in this series, *Supporting Relationships and Friendships*, gives plenty of good ideas.

Being bored or feeling relaxed

✎ Take some time now and write the difference between being bored and having a relaxing day:

....
....
....
....

List here how you feel and what you do and don't do when you are having a relaxing day:

....
....
....
....

List here how you feel and what you do and don't do when you are bored:

....
....
....
....

✎ Does the service user have days when he is relaxing?   Yes/No
✎ Does the service user have days when he is bored?   Yes/No

If you have answered 'Yes' to the service user having days when he is bored, what can be put in place to prevent the service user being bored?

....
....
....
....

MEETING THE NEEDS OF SERVICE USERS

On the next few pages you will read various exercises which, when completed, will tell you many things, mainly what the service user has or has not got in his life and his needs.

Exercise 1: Roles and responsibilities

We all need to be needed, both in and outside of work. To feel needed, we need to be able to fulfil roles, which give us responsibilities, no matter how large or small. We need to have realistic responsibilities that we can achieve.

✍ What is your role and what are your responsibilities in your own house? What is the service user's role and responsibilities in his own house?

Examples: parent, partner, cook, gardener, carer, window cleaner, teacher, breadwinner, etc.

....

....

....

What did this exercise tell you?

....

....

....

....

Did it tell you that the service user has few or no roles and responsibilities? Yes/No

Did it tell you that the service user had too many or too few responsibilities? Too many/too few

Exercise 2: How do you know what the service user wants or needs?

The answer is that you don't know what the service user needs. To answer this you could ask him and you could also use a model like Maslow's 'Hierarchy of Needs'. This is a theory in psychology that Abraham Maslow proposed in his 1943 paper 'A theory of human motivation'.

As you can see, it has five levels to it.

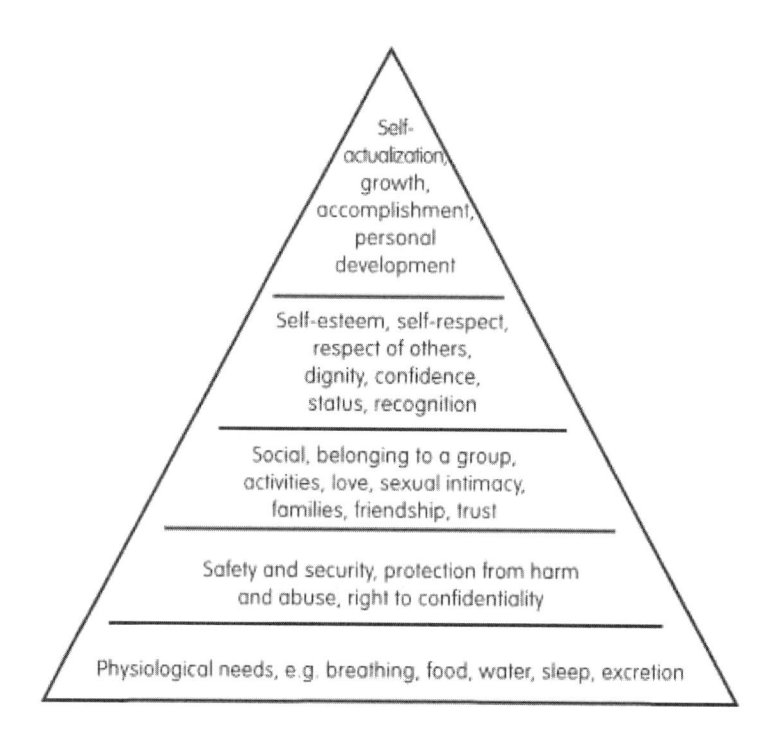

```
                    /\
                   /Self-\
                  /actualization,\
                 / growth,         \
                / accomplishment,   \
               / personal            \
              / development           \
             /_____ \
            / Self-esteem, self-respect,\
           /  respect of others,         \
          /   dignity, confidence,        \
         /    status, recognition          \
        /_____\
       /  Social, belonging to a group,     \
      /   activities, love, sexual intimacy, \
     /    families, friendship, trust         \
    /_____\
   /  Safety and security, protection from harm \
  /    and abuse, right to confidentiality       \
 /_____\
/ Physiological needs, e.g. breathing, food, water, sleep, excretion \
```

According to Maslow, until the two bottom lines are achieved, it is unlikely that you can move up and develop. Therefore, you need to look at how you can provide the service user with the right support before they can achieve the other levels or sections and reach self-actualization (assuming these have not been reached yet).

✎ Looking at Maslow's Hierarchy of Needs, which are being met in your place of work?

. . . .

. . . .

. . . .

A Community Care Assessment could assist in identifying some care needs and this may cover only the first two stages. *How to reach the other stages*:

- *Personal development and growth*: staff to enable the service user to learn new things and achieve. This can be anything from learning to prepare a snack, vacuum a carpet, swim, read or write to learning how to catch a bus, to getting a job, watering the plants or participating in a reminiscence group etc.

- *Status, recognition*: we all need a role or two and when we carry out these roles people thank us and appreciate us. By completing the roles and responsibilities exercise on pp.62–63 you will have seen if the service user has any roles and/or responsibilities where he lives. If the service user has not got any you may wish to discuss with him about bringing one or two in to start with. It can be large or small, e.g. clearing the table after a meal or taking their own crockery to the kitchen, or taking it in turn to chair the house meeting etc.

- *Social – belonging to a group*: staff within the home need to provide support to enable the service user to be in a group (if the service user wants to). Examples of being in a group can be anything from doing voluntary work to playing in a pool team in the pub, to joining a knitting circle, playing cards or dominoes group or a reading circle or working on an allotment.

- *Social – activities, love and friendship*: you will see by completing some exercises later in this workbook what the service user does during the day or evening and if he has friends etc. We all need to have friends and we all need to be loved. You may find the workbook *Supporting Relationships and Friendships* useful.

✎ If your place of work is not supporting service users to meet any of the levels in the diagram, what can you do about it?

. . . .

. . . .

. . . .

. . . .

SUPPORTING POSITIVE BEHAVIOUR

Exercise 3: How you spend your day

✎ Choose a day when you are off duty and complete the right-hand column. Then choose a day when you were on shift and complete the left-hand column with or for the service user.

Time	Service user	Me
1–3am		
3–5am		
5–7am		
7–9am		
9–11am		
11am–1pm		
1–3pm		
3–5pm		
5–7pm		
7–9pm		
9–11pm		
11pm–1am		

✎ Now you have completed this, what does it tell you?

....
....
....
....

Does it tell you:

- You had more 'freedom' than the service user to make choices   Yes/No

- You were able to decide what you wanted to do when you wanted to do it   Yes/No

- The service user was restricted in what he was able to do through:

    ○ lack of choice   Yes/No

    ○ timing of staff shifts did not allow service user to do things after 9 or 10pm.   Yes/No

Exercise 4: Daily activities

✎ By completing this exercise it will show you the activities the service user does during different parts of the day and week.

Day	Sun	Mon	Tues	Wed	Thurs	Fri	Sat
Morning							
Afternoon							
Evening							
Night							

✎ Now you have completed the chart, what does it tell you?

. . . .

. . . .

. . . .

. . . .

Can you see any problems with the service user's pattern of activities? What can you do about this?

. . . .

. . . .

. . . .

. . . .

Now you have completed these exercises you should have an idea about what the service user does during the day or the week. Also, ask the service user's family and friends and put together a person-centred plan which focuses on the individual service user.

GOING OUT

You may be concerned about a service user showing challenging behaviour while he or she is out and you will need to discuss with the service user and other relevant people such as your manager and the service user's family on how the behaviour can be prevented or reduced. The risk assessment should show how to reduce or prevent this behaviour.

Here are four case studies; you will find possible solutions to these following the case studies.

Case study 1: Jeffrey

Jeffrey is an adult with a learning disability who goes shopping once a week with staff on a Thursday, which is his choice of day to go. It is very crowded and he comes back angry and begins shouting.

✐ What does this tell you and what can be done about it?

....
....
....
....

Case study 2: Sally

Sally is a person with dementia, is hard of hearing and lives in a residential setting. You and your colleague walk up to Sally with a stand aid and ask her if she would like to go to the toilet. She is startled as she is approached by the two staff and the stand aid. You ask her again if she would like to go to the toilet and everyone is looking at her and she is getting embarrassed and angry.

✐ What does this tell you and what can be done about it?

....
....
....
....

Case study 3: Joe

Joe is a person with a mental health need. He lives in a hostel and needs support, especially in relation to hygiene – he does not wash regularly. He likes to go out to the local café but is often turned away as the staff there say he is too dirty to be in their café. This upsets Joe and he throws crockery. This has led the owners to threaten to call the police if he does not leave the café immediately.

✎ What can you do to enable Joe to go into the café?

....
....
....
....

Case study 4: Beryl

Beryl enjoys going out with staff. When she is out, she tries to run across the road in front of the cars. Staff have informed the manager of this and also that just one staff supporting Beryl is not enough, but the manager says that Beryl has a right to go out.

✎ What can be done to make it safe for Beryl to go out?

....
....
....
....

POSSIBLE SOLUTIONS TO THE CASE STUDIES

Case study 1: Jeffrey

Choose the least busy time of the day on the Thursday for Jeffrey to go shopping.

Case study 2: Sally

Staff can keep a small clear photograph of a toilet in their pocket and show Sally and raise five fingers to show they will be back in five minutes.

Case study 3: Joe

Joe needs to understand that it is his personal hygiene, i.e. lack of washing himself and his clothes, that the staff at the café are unhappy about, it is not him. There could be many reasons why Joe does not wash, e.g. he does not have the money for toiletries or he does not know how to use the washing machine. You could discuss with Joe a training programme on how to keep himself clean.

Case study 4: Beryl

The manager needs to know why more than one member of staff is needed and, once the manager understands this, will agree to increase staffing to two for a period of time. A risk assessment will need to be completed and a programme can be devised for all staff to follow, from the time Beryl leaves the house to the time she gets back and it should include that each staff member will stand either side of Beryl. If Beryl tries to run into the road, the staff members can stop her doing this.

Staff will need to follow the programme closely and be consistent as to what they ask Beryl to do. If they are not consistent, Beryl will get different messages, get confused, possibly angry and not learn to avoid running out in the road. Beryl could also be taught the dangers of the road by using books from the library, programmes from the Internet etc.

Staying in

Some staff think that to show they have done a 'good job' they encourage the service users to go out all the time. Staying in is also important as long as the service user is doing things that he likes, e.g. having time to watch DVDs or listen to his favourite music, doing housework, having friends round, sitting in the garden on a sunny evening etc.

> A good balance of going out and staying in because the service user wants to go out and stay in is fine.

The Principles of Care

Respecting Service Users with Challenging Behaviour

We all deserve to be treated with respect, and it is important to remember this when working with service users with challenging behaviour. It is essential that, even when presented with difficult behaviour, you provide the principles of care at all times.

RESPECT

It is important to be respectful to service users. This is partly having a respectful attitude, but also relates to the language you use. You should call the people you support by their preferred name: the name the person chooses to use. If you meet a service user for the first time and his records say Mr Terry Smith, do not automatically call him Terry. Ask him what he likes to be called: he may say he likes to be called 'Mr Smith', and if he does then make a note of this so all staff will call him Mr Smith. It is important that you listen to what the service user is saying at all times and show regard and courtesy. This will build trust and confidence and raise the service user's self-esteem.

PRIVACY

Everyone has a right to privacy, and you should respect the service user's right. For example, if you know some confidential information about a service user, ensure you keep it confidential. Sometimes, there will be times when the service user wants to be alone – perhaps when listening to music or when on the toilet. Being respectful of privacy will help to build trust.

There should be a private area where the service user can receive visitors. Some may like to receive visitors in their bedroom but many may like a different private area – one where others cannot intrude, like a private room. It is important that neither you nor or anyone else listen in on service users' conversations.

Remember to knock on the bedroom door before entering, and to avoid going into their bedroom if the service user is not in there – always get permission to enter.

An important point to make is that respecting privacy is not the same as simply leaving someone alone for long periods of time. Some service users may not be able to move easily, so need to be visited regularly to find out if they need any support.

If you are working in someone's home, remember to knock on the front door, or when using the key safe system, call out and announce yourself. Also, knock on the door when entering or re-entering a room inside the house. Remember it is the person's own home.

✍ What feelings do you think you would have if you needed a social care worker to visit you in your own home to deliver care?

....
....
....
....

EMPOWERMENT

Empowerment is all about giving the service user choices and the power to make the decisions they want. Within your role, you will enable the people you support to do as much as they can for themselves. This will provide the people you support with a sense of competence and confidence.

INCLUSION

This means ensuring that all service users are included and that nobody is left out. It is likely that sometimes you will need to assist service users in order to make sure that they can be included in activities and decision making. One example of an activity that may require support would be attending college.

INDIVIDUALITY

It is important to see the people you support as service users with their own strengths, needs, wishes and dreams. Each person will develop a sense of identity and this can be achieved by recognizing the preferences and likes of the person. An example could be supporting individuals to decorate their personal space the way they want to and this will reflect their own taste. Another way is to remember the person's special interest and support them if required to follow these interests.

INDEPENDENCE

Encouraging the people you support to do things for themselves is very important and you may need to give time for this to be achieved. You may feel that you are doing service users a favour by doing everything for them but by doing this you will reduce the service users' self-worth and self-esteem and prevent them from progressing, developing or maintaining their current skills.

DIGNITY

It is important to ask service users who they would like to support them with their personal care, whether this is in a residential setting or in a person's own home. The service user's culture may say that it has to be the same sex; female service users may prefer a female to support them. Some organizations have a policy that only same-sex staff will support the service users with their personal care.

When I have asked trainees about women's preferences about who assists them to bathe, they are usually able to tell me about women who share particular religions or cultures having common preferences – but remember, we are all individuals, and will have our own personal preferences.

Personal care should be carried out discreetly to avoid humiliation and embarrassment; a service user may refuse to receive any kind of support if you humiliate and embarrass him or her.

Here is an example of what you must *not do*:

Talk loudly to your colleague who is at the end of the hall, e.g.

'Mr Smith has just been toileted…'

'Mr Smith has just been fed…'

'Mr Smith has been hitting again…'

As with being respectful, how you speak has an effect on a service user's sense of dignity, so do think about what you say. Dignity gives the person self-worth and affords respect.

I was once told by a carer who used to work in a home supporting older people that dignity, respect and privacy can deteriorate and be neglected if staff think that the service users will not complain.

✍ Are dignity, respect and privacy regarded as important in your workplace?   Yes/No

If you have answered 'No' what can you do about it?

....

....

HUMAN RIGHTS

With the Human Rights Act 2000 in place, we can seek help if we feel that our human rights are being infringed. The Human Rights Act gives us the following legal rights:

- life
- freedom of slavery, servitude and forced or compulsory labour
- freedom from torture and inhuman or degrading treatment or punishment
- freedom of expression
- right to marry and have a family
- a fair and public trial within a reasonable time
- liberty and security of person
- freedom from retrospective criminal law and no punishment without law
- freedom of thought, conscience and religion
- respect for private and family life, home and correspondence
- freedom of assembly and association
- the prohibition of discrimination in the enjoyment of convention rights
- access to an education
- peaceful enjoyment of possessions and protection of property
- free elections
- not to be subjected to the death penalty.

The people who you support have often been denied some of the rights that they are entitled to; these rights are enshrined in national and international law, and you can promote these rights by advocating on behalf of the service user and by challenging any discriminatory practice or behaviour. There may also be an independent advocacy service in the area which the people you support should be made aware of.

EQUAL OPPORTUNITIES

Everyone should have equal access to services regardless of age, race, gender, disability, sexuality and culture.

PARTNERSHIP

It is important to work in partnership with the service user and others to achieve aims and goals. By working together you can share responsibilities and decision making and gain views and opinions. This makes the most of resources and values everyone's knowledge and skills.

CHOICE

Service users should choose and express their preferences e.g. what to eat, what to wear, where you want to live etc. You need to offer choice, and support the service users to take as much control over their own lives as is possible. Not only does this promote independence but also it raises the person's self-esteem. Not to have choices or to have them stopped suddenly can cause loss of confidence and low self-esteem.

If the service user is able to make choices you will need to enable him to know the consequences of making these choices. You need to know the person you are supporting and his level of comprehension: if he has never been given choice before, he could become worried or anxious not knowing what you are asking of him. Also, if he knows what choice is but has been given too many choices, then this could have the same effect. Speaking personally, I always become a little worried when I go into a cake shop and I am in a queue; there are too many cakes to choose from and I am very aware of the people waiting behind me. If they only had two cakes for me to choose from I would feel better and would be able to choose from just two items.

You can support the service user to make choices by:

- communicating in a way that the service user can understand
- not giving too many choices if it will upset and/or confuse the service user
- explaining and discussing the choices available and the consequences of those choices.

If the service user is discouraged from making choices he can become:

- angry
- withdrawn
- dependent on you.

BALANCING CHOICE WITH RESTRICTIVE CHOICE

Promoting choice is very important. However, there is another side to choice and that is *restrictive choice*. This is where it is in the service user's best interest to have choice and freedom restricted. If restrictions are present they must be recorded in the service user's support plan. These restrictions must be made by a multidisciplinary team.

> The plan describes any restrictions on choice and freedom [agreed with the service user] imposed by a specialist programme [e.g. a treatment programme for drug or alcohol misusers]; for mental health service users, in accordance with the Care Programme Approach and in some instances the Mental Health Act 1983. (CQC Care Home for Adults Standard 6)

> Where the service user is on the Care Programme Approach or subject to requirements under the Mental Health Act 1983, the service user's plan takes this fully into account. (CQC Care Home for Older People Standard 7)

✎ Please ask your manager if any of the people you are or will be supporting have any restrictions in place and the reasons for these.

Some service users will be able to make choices, others may not. It is wrong to assume that if someone has dementia or a learning disability, they cannot make any kind of choice.

> Some people with a learning disability may have been in long-stay institutions for most of their lives and not been offered choice before.

MAKING CHOICES: THE MENTAL CAPACITY ACT 2005

Under the Mental Capacity Act 2005 a service user has the right to make an unwise decision unless he lacks capacity and this applies if the decision is an everyday one or a life changing one.

The Mental Capacity Act provides a framework to protect the people you support in making choices and decisions. You may have a copy of this Act in your workplace and it will tell you what you should do; for example, in relation to assessing capacity, you should assume that the person has the capacity to make a decision unless proved otherwise. It also gives information on what should be done if a person lacks capacity. Remember that determining capacity means at the time the service user is making the decision.

If there is not a copy of the Mental Capacity Act 2005 in your workplace, you will be able to view it on the Internet. The Act has pages of information on how to ascertain if the people you support can make decisions.

✍ Please have a look at a copy, in particular sections on:

- Five key principles
- Independent Mental Capacity Advocate (IMCA)
- The making of 'living wills'
- The new criminal offence of ill treatment or neglect
- The new Mental Capacity Act Deprivation of Liberty Safeguards.

Deprivation of Liberty Safeguards

The Deprivation of Liberty Safeguards is often shortened to DoLS and is also known as the Bournewood Safeguards. DoLS applied to all care homes and hospitals from 1 April 2009. DoLS has its own Code of Practice although the Mental Capacity Act 2005 Code of Practice still applies.

As the title of the Act suggests, the Deprivation of Liberty Safeguards is about not depriving the people you support of their liberty or freedom. The people you support should have freedom to choose, including what they want to do, to wear and to eat, where they want to live, how they follow hobbies and interests, when they see family and friends etc.

An easy-to-read version of the Deprivation of Liberty Safeguards can be found on the Department of Health website: www.dh.gov.uk/en/Publicationsandstatistics/Publications/PublicationsPolicyAnd Guidance/DH_091868 or from www.publicguardian.gov.uk

Please note that at times the Mental Health Act 1983/2007 overrides the Mental Capacity Act 2005 and vice versa. For example under the Mental Health Act a service user may have his liberty (freedom) restricted because he is sectioned under the Mental Health Act. Under the Mental Capacity Act 2005 it would be unlawful to restrict a service user of his freedom.

People most likely to be affected by the Deprivation of Liberty Safeguards are elderly people with dementia, people with learning disabilities and others who lack the capacity to give consent on receiving treatment and/or care.

Health, Safety and Risk

There may be risks attached to what the service user wants to do because of his behaviour, e.g. he would like to go to the football match but gets angry because he does not like crowds.

THE IMPORTANCE OF RISK ASSESSMENTS

The Management of the Health and Safety at Work Regulations 1999 requires risks to be assessed in all areas of your work. Risks to the people you support, yourself and other people must be risk assessed. Your organization has a legal obligation to ensure the health and safety of service users and staff by identifying hazards and putting control measures in place to reduce risks and this includes any behaviour that could harm.

Domiciliary Care Standards

12.2: The risk assessment includes an assessment of the risks for service users in maintaining their independence and daily living within the home.

12.3: The manner in which the risk assessment is undertaken is appropriate to the needs of the service user and the views of the service user and their relatives are taken into account. The risk management plan is implemented and reviewed annually or more frequently if necessary.

12.7: Only staff who are both trained to undertake risk assessments and competent to provide the care are assigned to emergency situations and where pressure of time does not allow a risk assessment to be undertaken prior to provision of the care or support.

CQC Care Home for Adults Standard

42.6: The registered manager ensures that risk assessments are carried out for all safe working practice topics covered in Standards 42.2.

HEALTH, SAFETY AND RISK

> **CQC Care Home for Older People Standard**
>
> **38.6**: The registered manager ensures that risk assessments are carried out for all safe working practice topics and that significant findings of the risk assessment are recorded.

Everyone should have the same opportunities in life, e.g. leisure, education or housing, regardless of whether they have challenging behaviour or not. Your role is to support service users to communicate their needs, wants and wishes and reduce the challenging behaviour.

As a professional you have a duty of care towards the people you support and this could cause conflict as the people you support also have the right to take risks. A duty of care means you must take reasonable care to avoid the service users being harmed and a risk assessment will need to be written if there are any risks.

> As a social care worker, you must respect the rights of service users while seeking to ensure that their behaviour does not harm themselves or other people. (GSCC Code of Practice Standard 4)

Your role is to enable the people you support to understand the risks associated with making choices. This does not mean that if there is a risk then the choice does not happen.

A risk is balanced against the benefits of it being taken. There are risks attached to almost everything we do: crossing the road, going to a night club, getting a bus, visiting the bank, meeting friends, having a relationship. This is no different for the people you support. If we did not take risks, we would not learn and develop and our opportunities in life would be limited.

THE POSITIVE SIDE OF RISK: SERVICE USERS MAKING CHOICES

We all need activities and goals in our lives. Within your role as a social care worker you will need to know how to support service users to make choices and decisions, identify activities and goals and play a role in enabling the service users to achieve them. Some service users will achieve them without your help. It will depend on the service user as to how much support the service user would like or may need.

Everyone has the right to choose what they want to do, where they go, what they wear, and so on, and they may be able to make these choices independently. Others may require some help, which can be offered by verbally discussing ideas or using different methods of communication (you can find out more about these methods in another workbook in this series, *Effective Communication*).

Risk assessments are a very important tool in enabling the people you support to make choices on what they wish to do. In the past people receiving care have been 'wrapped up in cotton wool' and not allowed to do anything that could have or has a hazard attached to it. The result is that the service user has not had the opportunity to develop and try new opportunities.

If the service user has challenging behaviour this should not in itself prevent the service user from doing things he wants to do. A risk assessment needs to be a fair assessment, focusing on the service user as a whole and not just on the challenging behaviour. If you focus just on controlling the behaviours, you are stereotyping and discriminating. You will also be stereotyping if you assume that a service user who smokes is going to set fire to the home.

The risk assessment will be completed with/for the service user and will highlight the hazards (triggers) and the control measures that should be put in place etc. The risk assessment should look at the areas on the flow chart on p.81.

RISK ASSESSMENT, RISK MANAGEMENT AND RISK COMMUNICATION

Risk assessment

Risk assessment is the process of looking for hazards: if they exist, look at the likelihood for this to cause harm to a person or damage to property. Then look at the severity of the harm or damage. Look to see what control measures you have in place. You can carry out a calculation (risk rating) of the severity of the injury or damage, multiplied by the likelihood that it is going to occur (for ease of use, low = 1, medium = 2, high = 3). This will indicate if you need to introduce new control measures.

Risk management

Risk management is the process of seeing if adding new control measures is financially viable. Imagine a pair of scales: on one side is the cost of introducing additional control measures and on the other is the risk rating. If the cost is too high for minimal reduction of risk, it is not viable to put the additional control measures in place.

Risk communication

Risk communication is where you communicate the findings of the risk assessment to staff so that they use the existing control measures and any additional control measures (Source: Robert Baines, Health and Safety Manager, Home Farm Trust, personal communication, 21 August 2009).

WHAT TO DO IF THE SERVICE USER MAKES A CHOICE THAT PRESENTS A RISK

Discuss with the service user about having a meeting and who to invite, perhaps the manager, a relative, social worker or advocate. Under the Mental Capacity Act a service user has the right to make an unwise decision unless he lacks capacity. The meeting will:

Look for hazards (triggers)
↓
Identify who or what might be at risk and how
↓
Assess the likelihood of the risk
↓
Identify ways to reduce these risks
↓
All of this will be recorded on a risk assessment form
↓
Date will be set for the risk assessment to be reviewed.

Recording

Risks must be recorded on a risk assessment form in areas where people are especially vulnerable (you can see a sample risk assessment form on p.84).

Review

After each incident your company has a legal duty to review all relevant risk assessments relating to the person or people involved and the tasks involved in the incident. Your manager will show you the revised risk assessments that will contain revised measures to combat any future situation and you will be asked to read them and sign the sheet or form to say you have read the revised guidelines.

Each time the risk assessment is reviewed it will show how the service user is progressing and developing. When this happens and the service user becomes confident in what they are doing then this support may be reduced, but it will depend on the service user and you will need to discuss this with the service user and your manager.

Management guidelines

It is important that a procedure is in place which should be followed and this procedure is often called 'management guidelines'. These guidelines may be written in with the risk assessment or separately. They will guide you through what you need to do when a service user is becoming anxious and/or challenging. The guidelines will have boundaries written into them, which will enable the service user and the staff to know what is acceptable and what is not acceptable.

You will come across numerous guidelines and you must follow them. Please do not change them by yourself as they will have been written by very experienced professionals, e.g. behavioural therapists, psychologists etc. If you feel that any area of the guideline should be changed, you should pass your comments on to your supervisor or manager where they can be discussed fully. Guidelines work only when everyone is following them and working the same way.

Your supervisor or manager will discuss the following areas with you:

- training needs
- dress code, i.e. what you can and cannot wear
- support plans
- risk assessments
- guidelines on what to do if a service user is challenging.

HEALTH, SAFETY AND RISK

DRESS CODE

It is advisable to dress appropriately for work; you should not wear:

- jewellery (except wedding ring and ear studs)
- hair or face jewellery
- exposed shoes such as sandals or ones with heels
- tight clothing.

Remove your glasses if safe to do so when supporting a service user who is anxious or wear glasses with bendy frames. You may wish to wear a watch that has an elasticized or Velcro strap, so you can quickly take it off if required.

IDENTIFICATION CARD

Most organizations provide identification cards for staff that work with people who have challenging behaviour. If anything happened when you were outside you could show people your ID card.

NAME BADGES

Most organizations provide name badges for staff. The advantages are that visitors know who staff members are and service users know who staff members are, especially if staff are visiting in the service user's own home.

The disadvantages are that if staff wear their name badges while out with the service user, it can draw attention to the service user, which can result in the service user becoming distressed.

SUPPORTING POSITIVE BEHAVIOUR

RISK ASSESSMENT FORM

PART 1 STOP	**EVENT SCENARIO:**
	DATE:
	LOCATION

PART 2 THINK	**Safety Assessment**		
	Tick hazards introduced to task and any other potential hazards created by task			
	Slips, trips or falls on the same level		Entry into a confined space	
	Falling from height		Dust	
	Falling/flying objects		Fumes	
	Heat/fire/explosion		Noise	
	Asphyxiation/drowning		Vibration	
	Risk to equipment		Electricity	
	Contact with stationary object		Radiation (ionising and non-ionising)	
	Object overturning/collapsing		Lighting	
	Manual handling		Temperature	
	Unsecured load		Adverse weather	
	Vehicles		Untested equipment	
	Risk to personnel from others (violence)		Risk to others	
	Others (specify):			

PART 3 ACT	Hazard and its Risk	Control Measures	Remaining Risk (low/med/high)

HEALTH, SAFETY AND RISK

PART 3 ACT	(tick appropriate box)	YES	NO	N/A
	Is the correct equipment available for the scenario?			
	Is a pre-brief necessary for staff?			
	Are all Staff adequately trained?			
	Are all personnel healthy to participate?			
	Further comments:			

PART 4 REVIEW	End of Event Review		
	1. Has the AIM been achieved?	Y	N
	2. Are there any training needs?	Y	N
	3. Has the scenario highlighted new hazards?	Y	N
	4. Has a de-brief been given?	Y	N
	5. Has all equipment been checked prior to being returned?	Y	N
	6. Have outcomes been passed to relevant department?	Y	N
	Further comments:		

Comments of the Assesor:

ORIGINAL ASSESSMENT					
Name:		Signed:			
Date sent to H & S Manager					
REVIEW DATE					
Date:	Date:	Date:	Date:	Date:	Date:
Initial:	Initial:	Initial:	Initial:	Initial:	Initial:

Reporting and Recording

As a social care worker you have a duty of care and a responsibility to report and record anything that affects the well-being of the service user and this includes challenging behaviour.

> Reporting is telling someone verbally what has happened.
> Recording is writing it down.

KEEPING RECORDS

What to do!

You must report and record all factual evidence. This means you report and record what you saw. You must sign and date what you have written and you are doing this to confirm that what you have written is correct.

> Written reports must be objective and not subjective, i.e. they must cover what happened and not your opinion on why it happened.

What not to do!

Please do not use whiting-out fluid. If you use this it could be said that evidence has been tampered with and will be invalid. If you make a mistake, put a line through it and initial it.

✍ Do you know where to put the confidential completed form?   Yes/No

If you answered 'No', please ask your manager.

If there is an incident, there will be records that you will need to complete. These may vary in different services but here are a few examples:

- ABC charts
- mood diaries and mood charts

- an incident/accident form
- a Regulation 37 form which should be sent to CQC (if you work in a registered workplace)
- the service user's file.

The service user may be asked to complete their own chart or form if they are able to.

ABC CHARTS

Each service user should have a chart to be completed when they have been anxious and challenging. This form is called Antecedent, Behaviour, Consequences chart (some shorten this and call it an 'ABC chart'). By recording what happened prior to, during and after the event, you will be able to identify why the incident happened and put a plan in place to reduce or prevent it happening again.

Each incident should be recorded separately, i.e. if another incident starts after five minutes of the previous one finishing, then this is another incident. The ABC chart enables you and the service user to record and monitor incidents involving behaviour. This enables discussion on the information on the ABC chart and learning how to prevent and/or manage incidents like this again.

The following chart will show you that you need to record:

- what the service user was doing before the incident
- details of the incident
- what the service user did after the incident.

By completing this chart for a period of time, e.g. two weeks, it will show:

- a pattern
- the frequency
- when it happened
- what the behaviour is
- who was involved.

This enables you to learn about the person, rather than just saying 'He's got challenging behaviour' (which unfortunately I hear all too often). It will enable you to identify a pattern of behaviour.

This will enable something to be put in place to prevent it happening again. You will see on the sample ABC chart a few examples and beneath it a few explanations on why the behaviour may have occurred.

Sample ABC Chart

Name of service user: _____ Review date: _____

Date and time	Before the incident	Details of incident	What the service user did afterwards	Signature of staff
	1. Sat on the settee	Member of staff walked in the lounge and changed the TV channel. Service user tipped the coffee table over and then cried	Ran to his bedroom	
	2. Service user was asked to help prepare the table for tea	Banged his head against the window and then screamed	Sat quietly at table waiting for his tea	
	3. Finished drinking his cup of tea	Banged his empty mug on the table	Had another cup of tea	

Explanations on why the behaviour may have occurred

1. Member of staff walked in the lounge and changed the TV channel, which upset the service user as he was watching the TV.

2. Service user did not want to help prepare the table for tea.

3. He banged his empty mug on the table to get another cup of tea.

Benefits from challenging

What is the service user getting from the behaviour that makes him want to do it again? For example, if a service user bangs his head and gets a cup of tea afterwards he will learn that banging his head is the right way to get a cup of tea and will continue to bang his head to get one. Having said this, if a service user has a headache he could bang his head and this could continue until you notice he has a headache and does something about it.

MOOD DIARIES AND MOOD CHARTS

Mood diaries and charts are another two methods of gathering information, this time on 'moods'.

They can record how the service user is feeling, how many hours sleep he has had (if he has a problem with sleeping, either not getting enough sleep or sleeping too long) and, where appropriate, list the medication that is being taken, stressful events etc. Recording the service user's weight weekly or monthly may also be needed.

Keeping these records will enable the GP to see if there is a pattern to the moods. Having it written down will enable the GP to understand it more easily rather than the patient trying to remember everything and perhaps forgetting the most important bits. It is best to complete it at the end of the day as you can reflect on the day and how you were feeling.

Here are a few examples of what can be used to record moods:

- Calendars: These are a good way of starting to record moods. They are easy to purchase in the shops and they come in different shapes and sizes. When choosing which one to buy the customer will need to consider the amount of space there is to write on it, how colourful and bright it should be (some people may prefer a clear black and white calendar with no pictures on as they could be a distraction, others may prefer it to be colourful as this could raise their spirits).

- Mood diaries and mood charts: These are another good way of recording moods and the layout can be as simple or complicated as you wish it to be.

- Diaries are easy to purchase and again it will depend on the type of diary you want; you will need to ensure that it has sufficient space for you to write in.

- You could devise a chart and put in the left-hand column whatever you want to record. A basic chart is shown below.

SUPPORTING POSITIVE BEHAVIOUR

Day/month	1st	2nd	3rd	4th	5th	6th	7th	8th	9th
Waking up									
After breakfast									
After medication									
Before lunch									
After lunch									
After medication									
Before evening meal									
After evening meal									
Before going to bed									
In bed									

Code:
A = angry   S = sad
CS = crying/sad   M = menstruating
H = happy   TS = trouble sleeping

Using a different coloured pen for each of the codes will enable the problem area show up. A suggestion for colours could be:

- orange for being happy
- red for being angry
- brown for being sad
- blue for menstruating.

Alternatively you may wish to use pictures or stickers, especially if it is for children or people who like or need pictures to see what is happening. This may enable the individual to participate in completing their own calendar, mood dairy or mood chart.

INCIDENT/ACCIDENT FORM

Below is an example of an incident/Accident form. This form will be completed each time there has been an incident or accident.

| ACCIDENT | | INCIDENT | | NEAR MISS | |

To be completed and signed in ALL CASES

DETAILS OF PERSON INVOLVED:

NAME:

Place of Work:

Employee ☐   Service User ☐   Other ☐   Date of Birth ☐

Job Title/Other

Address:

DETAILS OF OCCURRENCE

Date and Time of Occurrence:

From the check list enter the code number against each of the following headings

Severity ☐   Accident Type ☐   Contributing Factors ☐
Location of Event ☐   Type of Injury ☐   Injured Part ☐
RTA ☐

Address of Occurrence:

Where if off Premise:

SUPPORTING POSITIVE BEHAVIOUR

To whom and time reported:	

Fully describe the occurrence and any treatment given:	

Please use another sheet if required

RIDDOR REPORTED (F2508)?	**YES**		**NO**		**DATE**	

Tick the appropriate boxes:

Remained at Work		First Aid		If booked off work how many days?	
Booked off Sick		Taken Home			
Attended A&E/GP		Taken to Hospital by Ambulance			

Name and Address of Witnesses:	
1.	2.

Date and Time Occurrence Reported:		

Signed...................... Name:....................... Date:........

Line Manager's Comments:	

Signed...................... Name:....................... Date:........
(Line Manager)

92

INCIDENT CHECKLIST

SEVERITY	ACCIDENT TYPE	CONTRIBUTING FACTORS
1. Absence from work for more than 3 days	1. Assault	1. Condition of Building
2. Amputation	2. Crushed	2. Condition of floor
3. Any penetrating injury to the eye	3. Collision with moving object	3. Deliberate action of other
4. Chemical or hot metal burn to the eye	4. Collision with stationary object	4. Deliberate action of Service User
5. Death	5. Electrocution	5. Drug/Alcohol abuse
6. Dislocation of the shoulder, hip, knee or spine	6. Equipment Failure	6. Enduring health condition
7. Fracture	7. Exposure to explosion	7. Obstruction
8. Hospitalised for more than 24 hours	8. Exposure to fire	8. Remove faulty equipment from use
9. Injury resulting from electric shock	9. Exposed to harmful substance	9. Temporary personal contact
10. Loss of sight (temporary or permanent)	10. Injury by an animal	10. Use of household equipment
11. Minor Injury	11. Manual Handling	11. Use of industrial equipment
12. Unconsciousness	12. Near Miss	
	13. Other kind of accident	
	14. Slip, Trip or Fall	

LOCATION OF EVENT	TYPE OF INJURY	INJURED PART	
1. Bathroom	1. Bruising	1. Head	19. Knee Rt
2. Bedroom	2. Burn/scald	2. Face	20. Knee Lt
3. Common room	3. Concussion	3. Eye Rt	21. Shin Rt
4. Craft room	4. Cuts	4. Eye Lt	22. Shin Lt
5. Dining room	5. Dislocation	5. Ear Lt	23. Ankle Rt
6. Front drive	6. Fracture	6. Ear Rt	24. Ankle Lt
7. Front garden	7. Graze	7. Neck	25. Foot Rt
8. Front steps	8. Irritation	8. Shoulder Rt	26. Foot Lt
9. Hallway	9. Pulled Muscles	9. Shoulder Lt	27. Upper arm Rt
10. Kitchen	10. Puncture Wound	10. Chest	28. Upper Arm Lt
11. Lounge	11. Scratching	11. Breast Rt	29. Elbow Rt
12. Office	12. Sprain	12. Breast Lt	30. Elbow Lt
13. Rear garden	13. Strain	13. Abdomen	31. Lower Arm Rt
14. Rear steps		14. Groin	32. Lower Arm Lt
15. Shed	**RTA**	15. Back Upper	33. Wrist Rt
16. Shower room	1. Trust vehicle	16. Back Lower	34. Wrist Lt
17. Stairs	2. Police involved	17. Thigh Rt	35. Hand Rt
18. Toilet	3. Staff member error of judgement	18. Thigh Lt	36. Hand Lt
19. Utility room	4. 3rd party error of judgement		
20. Workshop	5. Insurance report attached		
21. Other (Please Describe)			

Reproduced with kind permission from Home Farm Trust

REGULATION 37 FORM

Care Quality Commission Regulation 37 Form
NOTICE OF DEATH, ILLNESS OR OTHER EVENT
(Regulation 37 of the Care Homes Regulations 2001)

Name and address of home:	Date of event:
	Name of any resident(s) involved:
	Name of any staff involved and job title(s):

Type of notification. Please tick appropriate box:

a) The death of any service user, including the circumstances of his/her death ☐

b) The outbreak in the care home of any infectious disease that, in the opinion of any registered medical practitioner attending persons in the care home, is sufficiently serious to be so notified ☐

c) Any serious injury to a service user ☐

d) Serious illness of a service user at a care home at which nursing is not provided ☐

e) Any event in the care home that adversely affects the well-being or safety of any service user ☐

f) Any medication error that required medical intervention ☐

g) Serious error involving controlled drugs ☐

h) Any theft, burglary or accident in the care home ☐

I) Any allegation of misconduct by the registered person or any persons who work at the care home ☐

Action taken by care home in response to event:
Signature of registered person making this notice:
Date:
FOR CQC USE ONLY
Description of any relevant circumstances:

Decisions

Tick the appropriate box and give reasons for the decision

Refer to Regulation Manager – urgent follow-up action indicated ☐

Refer to Regulation Manager – follow-up action indicated ☐

No further action needed ☐

Reasons: ....

....

Signature: ....

Date: ....

Random inspection needed ☐

Other follow-up action needed (specify) ☐

....

....

....

Follow-up needed at next key inspection ☐

Signature: .... Regulation Manager

Date: ....

Logged as event on R&I System

By: .... Date: ....

✐ Please ask your manager where the accident/incident/near miss forms or book are kept and also who has the responsibility to inform the Care Quality Commission via the Regulation 37 form.

Support plan

Support plans were mentioned earlier on pp.55–58. Each organization will have its own designed support plan.

✎ If you have not seen one yet, please ask your manager if you can have a look at one and write the date here.

CONFIDENTIALITY

✎ Some staff may not understand exactly what confidentiality means and therefore may not report behaviour because it is confidential to the service user. Please now discuss with your manager what the meaning of confidentiality is and write your understanding of it here:

....

....

....

Taking Care of Yourself and Being Supported

Working with service users who are expressing themselves through behaviour can be very tiring, especially if the person is challenging for a prolonged period. If at any time you feel you need to leave the area and have some space or 'time out', you should discuss this as soon as is practicable with your senior or manager. It is a strength to do this and a period of 'time out' may be given when appropriate. The senior or manager may not be able to give you 'time out' there and then but should be able to arrange for another staff member to replace you shortly.

It is important that you and others who have been involved in incidents, including service users, or have witnessed incidents have an opportunity to talk through the incident and reflect, e.g. discuss what you did and if it helped the situation by de-escalating it or did it make it worse? This is sometimes called a debrief.

The service user who has been challenging should also be offered the opportunity of discussing the incident. You need to give time for the service user to be ready to discuss his behaviour and the reasons why he showed it. Please be aware that the service user will, more than likely, feel very embarrassed about what he has done. You must not blame the service user for what he did; instead you must listen to what he has to say and then discuss with him how he could have done things differently.

If after the event you are experiencing difficulty, i.e. stress or unease about working with service users please discuss it with your supervisor or manager. In the event of these two being off duty, you can discuss it with another senior member of staff, who will be happy to talk through the situation with you.

You will receive a minimum of six meetings per year and these are called supervision meetings or one-to-one meetings with your supervisor or manager. This will give an opportunity to do the following:

- Reflect on your practice, things that have gone well and things that have not gone well, e.g. perhaps you were following the behavioural guidelines and it did not go as planned; there are several reasons why this could happen, e.g. the service user has shown a new behaviour, and/or the guidelines need receiving or you require more training etc.

- Discuss areas of achievement for both the service user and yourself.
- Consider any issues that may be present.
- Receive feedback on your role.

> Practice can be reviewed in a supervision or one-to-one meeting or in a clinical group supervision: it will depend on the type of organization you work in as to which one you will receive.

WHAT SUPPORT WOULD I LIKE MY MANAGER TO OFFER ME?

When reading this question, you may feel that you do not need support. We all need support. The Government Task Force on violence to social care staff is placing a greater emphasis on support after a violent incident which results in physical or emotional harm to a staff member. Your workplace must give prominence to the provision of debriefing, counselling and other forms of support. This can be done only if you will inform people about what support suits you.

✎ I would like my manager to give me the following support:

....

....

....

Exercises

Below are some exercises that you can discuss as part of a supervision session and should help you to reflect on your work:

✎ Exercise 1: If someone is challenging or self-harming, to ensure safety for each service user, should they be discouraged until they are calm before they:

- have a bath (if they want one)
- go shopping or to the pub

- be left alone
- be supported on a one-to-one staff ratio in their bedroom?

If you were worried about going out with the service user, could another member of staff come with you?   Yes/No

✍ Discuss how you have felt prior to, during and after an incident:

....
....
....

Ask what you should do following an incident, e.g. should you:

- discuss it with the service user
- carry on as though nothing has happened?

Discuss what you would do if you were worried about being with him. Think about how a service user would feel if you did not follow his behavioural guidelines.

✍ Exercise 2: Discuss with your supervisor the following items:

- an incident you have witnessed or supported
- what you did
- what worked well
- what did not work well
- what you can do, if needed, to be more effective next time.

✍ Exercise 3: Think about why you are supporting people who have challenging behaviour.

It is important that you are working with people who have challenging behaviour for the right reasons and not because you want to have power or control over the service users' lives.

Why do I support people who may challenge? (Please tick where appropriate.)

- They need me
- I am strong enough to stop them challenging. If so, how?
- It makes me feel powerful, I am in control
- I understand their anxieties and can support people through it

TAKING CARE OF YOURSELF AND BEING SUPPORTED

- I like the 'buzz' it gives me
- I like to feel 'big' and 'brave' so I can tell my mates down the pub
- I am a woman, I can cope
- I am a man, I can cope
- I feel the job is worthwhile
- I feel really sorry for them

✍ After you have completed the above exercise, please show your manager.

Have you discussed the above exercises with your manager?   Yes/No

What do you think are the feelings or stress prior to, during and after a challenging situation that you may have?

....
....
....

How will you manage these?

....
....
....

How will you support a colleague prior to, during and after a challenging situation?

....
....
....

TRAINING

It is important that all staff receive training on how to support the service user. If you are supporting service users who present challenging behaviour, you should receive training on:

- principles of care
- person centred planning which puts the service user at the centre of the planning e.g. finding out what is most important to the service user, what his wants and needs are and how to get these things met

- effective communication
- risk assessment training (if applicable to your role and the position you hold)
- specific training on how to implement strategies that will reduce the behaviours over time for specific service users
- physical intervention procedures and techniques (if applicable):

Staff should receive training in the wider implications of restraint (including legal issues) and the different types of restraint.

Training should be provided in the area of equality and diversity to help recognize particular issues regarding a person's race, gender including gender identity, sexual orientation, disability, age, religion or belief.

Training should be based on an audit of the specific needs of the people being supported, and tailored to address these identified needs.

Staff should not receive training in unacceptable restraint methods as this could legitimize restraint that should not be used in any circumstances. e.g. Restraint that relies on the direct infliction of pain.

Any staff using planned physical intervention must have had appropriate training in its use.

Physical interventions training delivered to staff who work with people with learning disabilities or an autistic spectrum condition should be from a source accredited by BILD (British Institute of Learning Disabilities). (extracted from CQC website)

Information on risk assessments and record keeping in relation to physical intervention (restraint) can be found on the CQC website, www.cqc.org.uk

Some homes put more staff on shift in the hope that this will decrease the challenging behaviour but if the support staff do not support the service users in a person-centred way, the service user can become upset and show this upset through behaviour.

> It is important that the whole staff team are trained to the same level to provide a consistent approach.

'Psychotropic medication may be very effective when there is an underlying psychiatric disorder but there is concern that too often this medication is used as an alternative to adequate staffing' (Department of Health 2001).

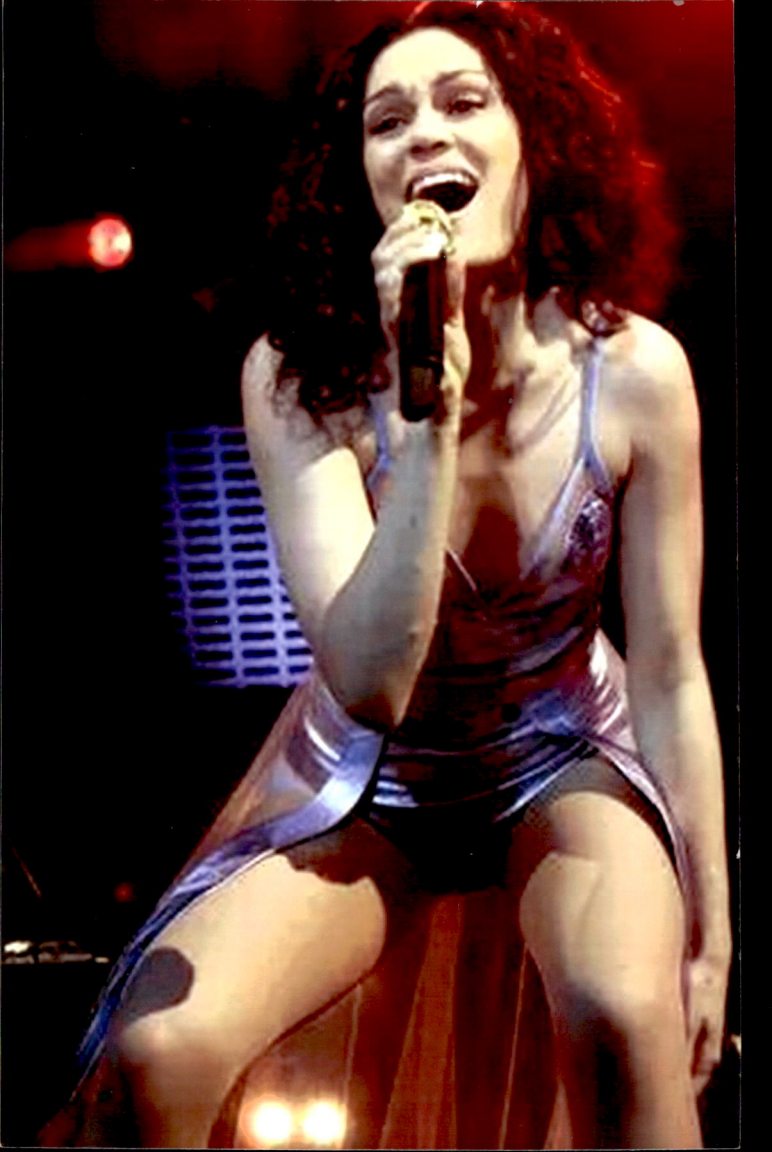

TAKING CARE OF YOURSELF AND BEING SUPPORTED

Do you remember this definition from p.15? Challenging behaviour is 'culturally abnormal behaviour of such intensity, frequency or duration that the person or others are likely to be placed in serious jeopardy or behaviour which is likely to seriously limit or delay access to and use of ordinary community facilities' (Emerson 1995, p.3).

✍ Are the service users stopped from going out because they have challenging behaviour?   Yes/No

If you answered 'Yes', what can you do about this?

....

....

You have nearly completed this book. Now try the 'knowledge' exercises below and check the answers with your manager.

✍ Exercises to check your understanding:

What does challenging behaviour mean?

....

....

Give four reasons why the people you support have challenging behaviour:

1. ....

....

2. ....

....

3. ....

....

4. ....

....

List two reasons why a service user may be upset with you or a colleague because he is angry and frustrated about something and what you can do about it:

1. ....

....

2. ....

....

SUPPORTING POSITIVE BEHAVIOUR

Give two examples of how you can establish contact and minimize the risk of the person becoming aggressive and/or abusive:

1. ....
   ....

2. ....
   ....

Give two examples of constraints to communication:

1. ....
   ....

2. ....
   ....

How would you support someone who had challenging behaviour?

....
....
....

What fears do you have when faced with a situation?

....
....
....

How does the service user feel after he has challenged the service?

....
....
....

How do you feel?

....
....
....

How do others feel?

....
....
....

What is the difference between being assertive and being aggressive?

....
....
....

Give two examples of how your own behaviour can affect others:

1. ....
....

2. ....
....

What do your organization's policies say about working with people with challenging behaviour?

....
....
....

How can you evaluate your own performance and competence when supporting people who have challenging behaviour?

....
....
....

How can stereotyping affect a risk assessment?

....
....
....

Self-Assessment Tool

I know how to communicate with each service user	Yes/No
I know where and how to stand when supporting each service user	Yes/No
I have read all service users' care plans	Yes/No
I know how to prevent service users challenging	Yes/No
I know what an ABC chart is and how to complete it	Yes/No
I know how to complete a health and safety form	Yes/No
I know how to complete a control and restraint form (if applicable)	Yes/No
I know how to complete the control and restraint book (if applicable)	Yes/No
I have received training on control and restraint supportive holds (if applicable)	Yes/No
I have received training on breakaway or blocking techniques	Yes/No
I have got an identification card	Yes/No
I am comfortable supporting service users who may challenge	Yes/No
I have attended health and safety training	Yes/No
I have read all the relevant risk assessments	Yes/No
I know how to dress appropriately for work	Yes/No

Signature of Learner . . . . Date . . . .

Signature of Supervisor . . . . Date . . . .

What one thing will you do differently as a result of completing this training?

. . . .

. . . .

. . . .

. . . .

Certificate

....
Name of company

THIS IS TO CERTIFY THAT

....
Name of learner

Has completed training on

Supporting Positive Behaviour

ON

....
Date

Name of Manager/Trainer ....

Signature of Manager/Trainer ....

Name of workplace/training venue ....

Date ....

This training has covered:
- Definition of challenging behaviour
- Causes of challenging behaviour
- Feelings and reactions prior to, during and after an incident
- Touch
- Physical intervention
- Responding to challenging behaviour
- Self-harm
- Responsibilities
- The principles of care
- How to minimize and/or prevent challenging behaviour
- Care plans and support plans
- Needs
- Risk assessments
- Management guidelines
- Reporting and recording
- Support
- Exercises to check your understanding
- Legislation

Legislation and Useful Websites

LEGISLATION THAT COULD BE APPLICABLE TO THE PEOPLE YOU SUPPORT

Care Standards Act 2000
This Act (CSA) provides for the administration of a variety of care institutions, including children's homes, independent hospitals, nursing homes and residential care homes.

Data Protection Act 1998
This Act protects the rights of the service user on information that is obtained, stored, processed or supplied and applies to both computerized and paper records; it requires that appropriate security measures are in place.

Health and Safety at Work Act 1974
This Act promotes the security and health, safety and welfare of people at work; this also includes individuals who you support.

Human Rights Act 2000
This Act promotes the fundamental rights and freedoms contained in the European Convention on Human Rights.

Mental Capacity Act 2005
This Act provides a clearer legal framework for people who lack capacity and sets out key principles and safeguards. It also includes the 'Deprivation of Liberty Safeguards' which aim to provide legal protection for vulnerable people who are deprived of their liberty other than under the Mental Health Act 1983. The Act came into effect in April 2009.

Mental Health Act 1983 as amended by the Mental Health Act 2007
This Act makes provision for the compulsory detention and treatment in hospital of those with mental disorder.

NHS and Community Care Act 1990
This Act helps people live safely in the community.

Safeguarding Vulnerable Groups Act 2006
The aim of this Act is to strengthen current safeguarding arrangements and prevent unsuitable people from working with children and adults who are vulnerable. It will change the way vetting happens. The first part of the Safeguarding Vulnerable Groups Act came into force in October 2009. There is a timeline for the implementation of the rest of it over five years. The Safeguarding Vulnerable Groups Act 2006 was passed as a result of the Bichard Inquiry arising from the Soham murders in 2002, when the schoolgirls Jessica Chapman and Holly Wells were murdered by Ian Huntley (a school caretaker).

Sexual Offences Act 2003
This Act makes new provision about sexual offences, their prevention and the protection of children from harm and sexual acts.

USEFUL WEBSITES

All the following websites were accessed on 16 January 2010.

Action on Elder Abuse
www.elderabuse.org.uk
Works to protect, and prevent the abuse of, vulnerable older adults.

Age Concern
www.ageconcern.org.uk
Promotes the well-being of all older people

Alzheimer's Society
www.alzheimers.org.uk
Leads the fight against dementia

Care Quality Commission
www.cqc.org.uk
Inspects and reports on care services and councils and is independent but set up by government to improve social care and stamp out bad practice

Change
www.changepeople.co.uk
Promotes equal rights for people with learning difficulties and provides information in accessible formats, making it easier to understand

Department of Health
www.dh.gov.uk
Provides health and social care policy, guidance and publications for NHS and social care professionals

General Social Care Council
www.gscc.org.uk
Sets standards of conduct and practice for social care workers and their employers in England

Mencap
www.mencap.org.uk
Mencap is the voice of learning disability and works with people with a learning disability to change laws and services, challenge prejudice and directly support thousands of people to live their lives as they choose

Mind
www.mind.org.uk
Mind is the leading mental health charity in England and Wales and works to create a better life for everyone with experience of mental distress

References and Further Reading

REFERENCES

Care Quality Commission (CQC) (2009) *Restraint: How to Move Towards Restraint-Free Care.* Available at www.cqc.org.uk/guidanceforprofessionals/socialcare/careproviders/guidance.cfm?widCall1=customWidgets.content_view_1&cit_id=2627, accessed on 16 January 2010.

Department of Health (2000a) *Domiciliary Care: National Minimum Standards* (Commission for Social Care Inspection Communication Standard). London: Stationery Office. Available at www.dh.gov.uk/prod_consum_dh/groups/dh_digitalassets/@dh/@en/documents/digitalasset/dh_4018671.pdf, accessed on 16 January 2010.

Department of Health (2000b) *Draft Guidance on the Use of Physical Interventions for Staff Working with Children and Adults with Learning Disability and/or Autism.* London: Department of Health.

Department of Health (2001) *Valuing People: A New Strategy for Learning Disability for the 21st Century.* London: Department of Health.

Department of Health (2003a) *Care Homes for Adults (18–65)* (Commission for Social Care Inspection Communication Standard). London: Stationery Office. Available at www.cqc.org.uk/guidanceforprofessionals/adultsocialcare/nationalminimumstandards.cfm

Department of Health (2003b) *Care Homes for Older People.* London: Department of Health. Available at www.dh.gov.uk/en/Publicationsandstatistics/Publications/PublicationsPolicyAndGuidance/DH_4005819

Department of Health (2008) *Mental Health Act 1983: An Outline Guide.* London: Department of Health. Available at www.mind.org.uk/help/rights_and_legislation/mental_health_act_1983_an_outline_guide, accessed on 16 January 2010.

Department of Health (2009) *Deprivation of Liberty Safeguards.* Available at www.dh.gov.uk/en/Publicationsandstatistics/Publications/PublicationsPolicyAndGuidance/DH_091868 or www.publicguardian.gov.uk, accessed on 16 January 2010. (An easy to read version.)

Emerson, E. (1995) *Challenging Behaviour: Analysis and Intervention in People with Learning Difficulties.* Cambridge: Cambridge University Press.

General Social Care Council (GSCC) (2002) *Codes of Practice.* London: GSCC. Available at www.gscc.org.uk/codes, accessed on 16 January 2010.

Kinmond, A.N. and Kinmond, K.S. (2006) 'Self-harm.' *Student BMJ* 14, 397–440. Available at http://archive.student.bmj.com/issues/06/11/editorials/400.php, accessed on 16 January 2010.

Maxlow, A.H. (1943) 'A theory of human motivation.' *Psychological Review 50*, 370–396.

McGill, P 1, The Tizard Centre, University of Kent at Canterbury

Mental Capacity Act 2005 Code of Practice Section 6[4]. Available at www.mind.org.uk/Information/Legal/OGMHA.htm.

Surrey Care association (2010) *Restraint Guidance.* Available from www.sitesetadmin.co.uk/surreycare/downloads/CSCI-RestraintGuidance.doc

FURTHER READING

Ball, T., Bush, A. and Emerson, E. (2004) *Psychological Interventions for Severely Challenging Behaviours Shown by People with Learning Disabilities.* Leicester: British Psychological Society. Available at www.bps.org.uk/downloadfile.cfm?file_uuid=4A51DB4D-306E-1C7F-B697-0FDC5CA88DC9&ext=pdf, accessed on 19 April 2010.

Care Quality Commission (CQC) *Restraint: How to Move Towards Restraint-Free Care.* Available at www.cqc.org.uk/guidanceforprofessionals/socialcare/careproviders/guidance.cfm?widCall1=customWidgets.content_view_1&cit_id=2627, accessed on 16 January 2010.

Department of Health (1999) *Code of Practice to the Mental Health Act 1983.* London: Department of Health.

Department of Health (2002) *Guidance for Restrictive Physical Interventions: How to Provide Safe Services for People with Learning Disabilities and Autistic Spectrum Disorder.* London: Department of Health. Available at www.dh.gov.uk/en/Publicationsandstatistics/Publications/PublicationsPolicyAndGuidance/DH_4009673, accessed on 16 January 2010.

Department of Health (2007) circular under section 7 of the Local Authority Social Services Letter (LASSL) Act 1970. They released guidance (with DfES) in July 2002 called *'Guidance for restrictive physical interventions. How to provide safe services for people with learning disability and autistic spectrum disorder'.* Staff working in social care have a duty of care towards the people they are supporting. *'Independence, choice and risk a guide to best practice in supported decision making'* London: Department of Health

Health and Safety Executive (HSE) (2000) *Violence at Work.* London: HSE. Available at www.hse.gov.uk/lau/lacs/88-2.htm, accessed on 16 January 2010.

National Institute on Mental Health Excellence (NIMHE) (2004) *Physical Restraint and Seclusion.* Available at www.publications.parliament.uk/jt200405/pa/jtselect/jtrights/15/1511.htm, accessed on 19 April 2010.

Office of Public Sector Information (OPSI) (n.d.) *The Human Rights Act 1998.* Available at www.opsi.gov.uk/ACTS/acts1998/uk/pga_19980042_en_1, accessed on 16 January 2010. (Article 3 prohibits 'torture and inhuman or degrading treatment'; Article 5 acknowledges that 'everyone has the right to liberty and that it should only be restricted if there is specific legal justification'; Article 14 outlaws 'discrimination of all types'.)